Mediterranean Diet for Beginners

Flavor Recipes for Lifelong Health and Weight Loss for Beginners

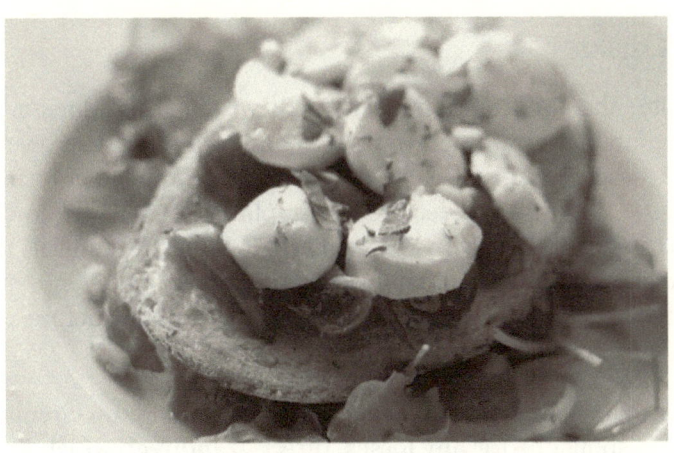

Table of Contents

Introduction

The surrounding lands of the Mediterranean Sea are the birthplaces of some of the most influential civilizations of the ancient world. For a very long period of time, it was considered the center of the world. Just think about it—the Egyptians, the Greeks, and then the Romans. The term Mediterranean was promoted by the Roman culture as it literally meant "inland," referring to the sea that was surrounded by the territories of the Roman Empire.

There are not many mentions of the conquered population adopting the cuisine of the conquerors—in this case, the Roman Empire—as the local cuisine mostly relies on the available ingredients. The Mediterranean Sea can play a vital influence not only over the climate of the surrounding lands but also on the local cuisine. The sea can provide plenty of fish while the surrounding lands are very fertile and favor crops like olives, grapes, wheat, and many others. People living in the surrounding lands of the Mediterranean Sea have preserved their way of life and what they eat, as every type of food is natural.

The concept of a Mediterranean diet was not invented by a Greek ancient philosopher or by a Roman senator. It wasn't even invented by the people of that age. In fact, it was theorized by an American scientist in the 1960s, and it started to gain more popularity in the 1990s. The main ingredients of the Mediterranean diet are vegetables, whole grains, fruits, fish, legumes (beans), and plenty of healthy fat. Plus, it also involves some moderate consumption of red wine. It's not a surprise that this diet started to become more popular in the 1990s as the American society was starting to experience the consequences of processed food, especially junk food. Of course, the American way of life involved too much sedentarism and too much junk food.

Too many diseases known to man are caused by the food we eat. Junk food is the main source of carbohydrates, which contain plenty of glucose, the body's default energy source. Unfortunately, when the glucose is not burned (this can happen through physical activity), it gets stored in your blood, raising the blood sugar and the insulin level. This is when the big problems start because it can lead to diseases like diabetes and other more severe diseases or conditions.

Some people consider AIDS as the disease epidemic of the twentieth century, but if you consider the number of people who are affected by diabetes, it's safe to consider it as the foremost disease of the previous century. The perspectives are also not too promising for the twenty-first century as this disease is growing at an incredibly fast pace.

So far, most people are aware that their current health condition is severely influenced by the food they consume, but unfortunately, not too many of them are keen on changing their diet and lifestyle. They only do so when the condition gets worse. Working out is definitely a way to improve one's health, but a healthy diet can have even more benefits on your health than physical exercise.

Most diets are focused on losing weight, and they suggest radical meal plans that are mostly deprived of nutrients, causing devastating effects on your body in the long run. That's why these diets are most likely to be broken, and when people do that, they mostly start to gain weight again. Such a temporary solution is not something to be tried at all.

A healthy diet should have positive effects on your body, not only when it comes to burning fat but also when it comes to preventing many diseases and health conditions. Also, it must not be too radical, as it should easily become a way of life, not something you try for one to two weeks and then quit for an undetermined period.

As there are many diets and alternatives claiming that they are the best for your body, you need to choose the right one for you. Some diets do not work because they are too radical. The more radical it is, the more likely people quit and start to gain weight. Since most diets involve restraining yourself from eating a certain type of foods, including the healthy type of food, they simply can't work in the long term. What you need for the long run is a well-balanced diet, which includes most types of natural food. You need to remember that more natural means healthier and more nutritious.

Natural food also tends to have a lower level of carbohydrates—meaning, less glucose. Processed food, like junk food, is calorie-dense but has little to no nutrient value. You get hungry very easily, and the worst part is that your body is craving for more, as it doesn't feel satisfying. On the other hand, natural food is known for covering your basic nutritional needs, so you feel less hunger. With a healthy diet, you don't have to worry about counting calories, as everything you eat is healthy. On top of that, you will most likely eat more fat than carbs, which means that you can switch the metabolic state of your body to ketosis when the body mostly runs on fat instead of glucose. During this state, your body can burn fat for energy, and your glucose level will lower as this state reactivates the insulin in your body. A perfect example of a diet that can turn your body into the fat-burning mode is the Mediterranean diet. This book is about its functionalities, benefits, and detailed meal plan to make everything clearer for you. So sit back and enjoy reading this book!

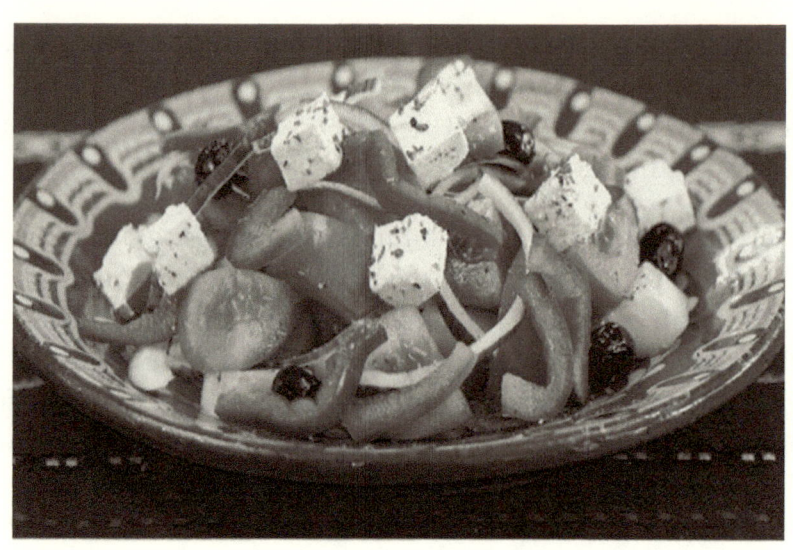

Chapter 1: Introduction to the Mediterranean Diet

There is no surprise that the Mediterranean diet is inspired by the healthy living habits of the people from the Mediterranean coasts (countries like Greece, Italy, France, and Spain). It can vary from region and country, and it can have different definitions, but it's all about eating high amounts of nuts, legumes, beans, fruits, vegetables, cereals, fish, grains, and plenty of unsaturated fats, like the olive oil. Also, it consists of lower levels of dairy products and meat (especially red meat). It has been associated with better health, especially a healthier heart.

The standard food pyramid divides the food into six different categories:

1. Fruits, salad, and vegetables

2. Rice, pasta, potatoes, bread, and whole-grain cereals

3. Cheese, yogurt, and milk

4. Nuts, beans, eggs, fish, poultry, and meat

5. Fats, spread, and oils

6. Food and drinks with high levels of fat, salt, and sugar

The Mediterranean diet, on the other hand, divided the food into four different categories. But at the base of the pyramid, we can find physical activity, something that people living in these areas are very keen on respecting. Above the physical activity level are the food categories, which represent the bulk of this diet.

1. The first food category in the Mediterranean diet pyramid is represented by the following: herbs and spices, legumes and seeds, beans, nuts, olive oil, grains (the vast majority represented by whole grains), fruits, vegetables.

2. The second food category is represented by fish and seafood. This level is also very important in this kind of diet.

3. In the third food category, you will find eggs, yogurt, cheese, and poultry.

4. The last food category of the pyramid is represented by sweets and meat.

This is similar to the standard food pyramid—the higher the level of the pyramid, the more unnecessary that food type is. Also, the most important drinks in this diet are water and red wine. Analyzing the Mediterranean diet pyramid, you will notice some key aspects of this diet:

- There is a high emphasis on the consumption of plant-based foods, like fruits, vegetables, legumes, whole grains, and also nuts.

- This diet encourages you to eat healthy fats, like canola or olive oil.

- Herbs and spices are preferred against salt when it comes to flavoring food.

- Fish or poultry is the meat of choice, not red meat, such as beef or pork.

- Moderate consumption of red wine is highly encouraged.

As you can see from the allowed food types, this diet doesn't mention anything about restrictions. You can consume each type of food mentioned above, depending on the necessity. The basic plant-based food should be consumed on a daily basis. Fish or poultry should be eaten at around twice a week. Yogurts or cheese should be consumed frequently but more moderately. Red meat and sweets should be rarely eaten. Eggs should be consumed on an occasional basis.

The Mediterranean diet is an LCHF (low-carb, high-fat) diet, which can mean plenty of benefits for your body. With all the abundance of processed food, eating more natural is a first step to improve your health. However, when you know how to balance the natural food intake, this is when the food can have even more results on your health and physical condition.

Nowadays, people's addiction to carbs should be treated a lot more seriously in our society. This addiction has caused too many diseases known today, and the best way to reverse this trend is to radically change your diet. Processed food is where carbs are mostly found. This type of food is calorie-dense but not nutrient-dense. It doesn't contain many nutrients, just a lot of carbs. This means that you will easily get hungry and your body will crave for this kind of food again.

Natural food is quite the opposite as it's more nutrient-dense than calorie-dense. It is more consistent than processed food, so you will not easily get hungry. The main purpose of healthy food is to make your body consume fewer carbs, which are the main sources for glucose, a substance that is normally the default "fuel type" for your body. But what happens when glucose is not burned completely (it rarely gets burned completely)?

Glucose will not remain forever to be burned during physical activity. The excess glucose gets stored in your blood, raising the insulin level and raising the blood sugar. Sounds familiar? Well, this is how diabetes starts. In order to reverse and prevent the accumulation of glucose, you have to train your body to run on something different, something like an eco-fuel type. This eco-fuel can be represented by fat, and the energy from fat can be obtained through the action of ketones.

You are probably wondering what ketones are and how they operate. Switching your meal type to have higher fat values will mean, first of all, glucose deprivation. In such a scenario, the body will start to look for different alternatives of fuel as the glucose level from your body is going down. The insulin level also lowers, which means that insulin gets reactivated and now is released to do its job, decreasing and regulating the blood sugar level.

When blood sugar goes down (at the same time with the insulin level), the ketone bodies multiply. Think of these ketones as some chemicals produced by your liver that are capable of breaking down the fat tissue and releasing the energy from there. The energy can be found in the fat reserves and in the fat you eat. Since the Mediterranean diet is rich in fats, it means that it encourages ketosis (the metabolic state associated with higher ketones and fat levels) and the keto-adaptation process (when the body is using fats as the default fuel type). Not only is this type of diet rich in fats, but most importantly, it's rich in unsaturated fats (olive oil is probably the best example of this type of fats).

The Mediterranean diet includes only healthy food, which can have plenty of health benefits over your body. All the ingredients can easily be found in supermarkets, which can provide you with everything you need for this diet. Also, the diet is not difficult or harsh like other diets. It's easy to follow as it doesn't involve lowering your meal size or the frequency of meals. You can have the main three meals of the day, plus snacks and desserts. What you need to do also is to associate the diet with physical exercise. Jogging, cycling, swimming, and working out at the gym are highly recommended in this case.

Some of you are probably asking, "Wait, didn't you say the Mediterranean diet is rich in fats? Shouldn't that get me fat?" That's not the case. As you favor your body to run on fats, it will only burn fats, and when you complement the diet with physical exercise, you just can't go wrong. This is why people living in the Mediterranean region are more healthy, fit, and agile. So far, it's obvious that this type of diet is low in carbs and high in fats. However, what's the protein level of it?

The diet doesn't encourage the consumption of fish, seafood, poultry, red meat, or eggs on a daily basis—meaning, it doesn't have a high protein level. Even though it's recommended to eat yogurts and cheese frequently (although in moderation), this still doesn't mean that you will get a high protein value in your food.

Proteins are also a source of glucose, and the nutritionists recommending this diet are also aware of that. A higher protein level may increase glucose intake, so your body can start running on glucose again. This is something that you need to avoid. The Mediterranean diet is not for bodybuilders as it is not the kind of meal plan that can favor muscle growth. However, it can still maintain your muscle mass at a more-than-decent level. Remember, physical exercise associated with this diet can still maintain your muscles even though the protein intake may not be satisfactory.

As you are about to discover in the following chapter of this book, the Mediterranean diet is one of the healthiest meal plans you can implement. It will help you eat better, and it also

15

has a positive impact on your health and on the weight loss process. It's really hard to think of a better balanced diet because this one seems to be the common ground for vegans, meat lovers, and keto diet fans.

The Mediterranean diet is among the meal plans with the most permitted ingredients. Such a dietary plan includes a plethora of available recipes that can be tried during this diet. You can easily choose from the available recipes and customize your meal plan according to your objectives. It can be practiced by almost anyone as no harm can come from following this diet. For incredible results, this diet should be regarded as a lifestyle, not something that is tried on a short-term basis. If you are following this diet, in the long run, you will notice that your body will start to lose weight.

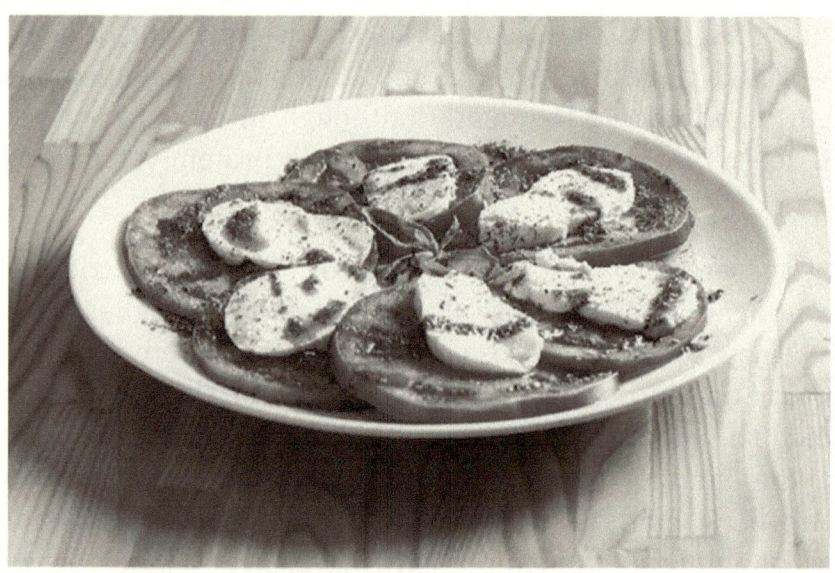

Chapter 2: Scientific Proof of Its Functionality

OK, so far, we have established what the Mediterranean diet is. But what are its benefits? Does it really work? There are plenty of diets and meal plans out there that claim they are the best possible diet, and they have impressive results when it comes to weight loss. Most diets focus on losing weight, and they present quick plans to achieve this goal in record time. However, are they healthy? The Mediterranean diet is keen on setting the right conditions for your body to become healthier, feel and look better, and also lose some weight. This meal plan happens to have plenty of benefits. Some of them are easily proven by scientific research, and others are not yet backed up by studies. Below, you can find the benefits proven by scientific research.[1]

Decreases the Risk of Frailty

Muscle loss and weakness are just symptoms of the frailty syndrome, which is more common in people with type 2 diabetes and in older people. There was a research published by the *American Journal of Clinical Nutrition* that discovered a higher reduction of frailty at people who consumed more

---

[1] Fernandez, Sonia. (2018) Top 5 Mediterranean diet benefits backed up by research. Retrieved from www.medicalnewsbulletin.com/mediterranean-diet-benefits-research/

vegetables, fruits, and alcohol. This led to the conclusion that there is a decreased risk of frailty in women with type 2 diabetes if they try the Mediterranean diet.

Lowers the Risk of Lung Cancer

Believe it or not, the Mediterranean diet has a positive effect when it comes to preventing terrible diseases such as lung cancer. The incipient studies related to the Mediterranean diet and lung cancer were conducted on fewer subjects and didn't have links to gender or types of lung cancer. "In a recent study conducted in the Netherlands, researchers investigated the association between the Mediterranean diet and the major lung cancer subtypes adenocarcinoma, squamous cell carcinoma, small cell carcinoma, and large cell carcinoma. They found that the risk of lung cancer was significantly reduced in both sexes where people had a high level of adherence to the diet. However, they do note that these findings may only be applicable to individuals with a normal body mass index (BMI) measurements. The study was published in the *British Journal of Nutrition*."

Substitutes the Most Common Treatments for Reflux

LPR (also known as the laryngopharyngeal reflux) is the result of the consumption of highly acidic food and drinks, activating pepsin (a stomach enzyme), which can cause serious damage.

Of course, the treatment for such condition is to balance the pH level by drinking alkaline water and eating low-acid food. Coincidence or not, the Mediterranean diet has enough alkaline to work as a cure, as shown by a research published in *JAMA Otolaryngology—Head & Neck Surgery*. This research was conducted on 184 patients, and it proved that there is a significant decrease in reflux symptoms for the patients following a Mediterranean diet compared to those on a regular diet.

Prevents and Fights against Muscle Loss

"Mediterranean diet benefits include a higher muscle mass in European women, thus protecting their health during old age. The study, published in the *British Journal of Nutrition*, found that a Mediterranean diet helps lower inflammation in participants. Inflammation is one of the main reasons for lowered muscle mass with age."

Decreases Your Blood Pressure

The Mediterranean diet consists of high levels of fats; but it also encourages the consumption of seafood, nuts, legumes, and the occasional red wine (red meat is extremely rarely consumed). All these food types play a regulating role when it comes to the blood pressure as they reduce the systolic blood pressure and enhance the blood function. All these are proven by a study published in the *American Journal of Clinical*

Nutrition that was applied to elderly people from Australia (at least sixty-four years old).

Research studies were also conducted on the people living in the Mediterranean basin, and the results were simply staggering. Among these people, the rate of heart diseases is incredibly low, and this is caused by the high-fat consumption (mostly olive oil). Their food is low in carbohydrates but extremely rich in polyunsaturated and monounsaturated fats, which can lower the level of triglycerides and LDL and increase the level of HDL cholesterol.

"In a detailed analysis within the Nurses' Health Study, trans fat from partially hydrogenated vegetable oils (absent in traditional Mediterranean diets) was most strongly related to the risk of heart disease, and both polyunsaturated and monounsaturated fat were inversely associated with risk. Epidemiologic evidence has also supported the beneficial effects of higher intakes of fruits and vegetables, whole grains, fish, and daily consumption of moderate amounts of alcohol. Together with regular physical activity and not smoking, our analyses suggest that over 80% of coronary heart disease, 70% of stroke, and 90% of type 2 diabetes can be avoided by healthy food choices that are consistent with the traditional Mediterranean diet."[2]

Sounds convincing enough! Well, that's because this diet has plenty of health benefits, even more than the ones mentioned above. More benefits can be found below:

---

[2] Willett, Walter. (2007). The Mediterranean diet: Science and practice. *Cambridge Core*. Cambridge University Press. Retrieved from www.cambridge.org/core/journals/public-health-nutrition/article/mediterranean-diet-science-and-practice/C383082DF00DDFE6475D0B8614EB0BE9

Enhances the Cognitive Function

Since the Mediterranean diet is packed with healthy fats, it can play a positive role in preventing cognitive decline and dementia. A study proved that 40% of the people on this diet showed lower risks of cognitive impairment.

Lowers the Risk of Heart Disease

There are several studies that demonstrate that the Mediterranean diet can lower the risk of cardiovascular diseases, including stroke, myocardial infarction (also known as a heart attack), and coronary heart disease. All these are made possible by the positive effect this diet has on cardiovascular risk factors like cholesterol, triglycerides, and high blood pressure.

Promotes Stronger Bones

There is a study that clearly emphasizes the effects of some compounds found in olive oil that may help preserve the bone density through the enhancement of maturation and proliferation of bone cells. Also, there is another study demonstrating that dietary patterns linked with the Mediterranean diet may prevent osteoporosis.

Controls Blood Sugar and Manages Diabetes

It's already known that a diet rich in fats can have a positive impact on the blood sugar and insulin level. The Mediterranean diet is a perfect example of a high-fat diet that is super healthy, so it has plenty of benefits for diabetes prevention. It can definitely prevent type 2 diabetes. It can also enhance the control of blood sugar and lower the cardiovascular risk for people who already have this disease.

There was a research in which this diet was compared to a low-fat diet. The study was conducted on people with type 2 diabetes. Those who followed the Mediterranean diet experienced better blood control and weight loss, and some of them didn't need diabetes treatment anymore.

Prevents Depression

So far, it's very clear what health benefits this diet has on a wide variety of people. Whether the impact is medical, mental, or physical, the Mediterranean diet is the kind of meal plan that can help you achieve that. The diet also has a positive impact from a psychological point of view as people on this diet may not experience depression. A study from 2013 showed that 98.6% of people following this diet have a lower risk of depression compared to those who were not following this diet very closely or at all.[3]

Protects against Cancer

Higher adherence to a Mediterranean diet may help fight off cancer. A systematic review of studies found that, overall, people who adhere to the diet the most have a 13% lower rate of cancer mortality compared to those who adhere the least. Specifically, these cancers include breast cancer, colorectal cancer, gastric cancer, prostate cancer, liver cancer, and head and neck cancer.[4]

If you think these are all the benefits of this diet, you couldn't be more wrong. Other benefits may include (some of them are not quite proven yet) the following:

1. *It has a better and healthier weight management system.* As you probably know, processed foods are not the consistent type—meaning, they don't cover your basic nutritional needs. They are very calorie-dense but low in nutritional value, not having too many nutrients besides carbs. You can easily

---

[3] University Health News. (2018). 6 major benefits of the Mediterranean diet. Retrieved from www.universityhealthnews.com/daily/nutrition/6-major-benefits-of-the-mediterranean-diet/

[4] University Health News. (2018). 6 major benefits of the Mediterranean diet. Retrieved from www.universityhealthnews.com/daily/nutrition/6-major-benefits-of-the-mediterranean-diet/

get hungry after consuming such food. On the other hand, the Mediterranean diet is rich in fiber and healthy fats. They can cover a lot better your basic nutritional needs, and you also feel more satiated after consuming such food. The fiber from this diet can improve your metabolism and can play a very important role in a healthy weight loss process.

2. *It can be good for your gut.* The bacteria resulted from the food you eat can cause serious damage to your guts or stomach. It's been proven that people on a Mediterranean diet have a higher concentration of good bacteria in their microbiome than people following a typical Western diet (processed or junk food). There are scientific studies that show that the consumption of food like legumes, fruits, or veggies can raise the good bacteria level by 7%.[5]

3. *It can extend your life.* Well, this is open to debate as the main idea is based on the life expectancy of the people from the Mediterranean basin. They live longer because they are following this diet, which may lead to better heart health and other medical benefits favorable for longer life.

---

[5] Laurence, Emily. (2019). 9 Mediterranean diet benefits that explain why experts love it so much. Retrieved from www.wellandgood.com/good-food/mediterranean-diet-benefits/

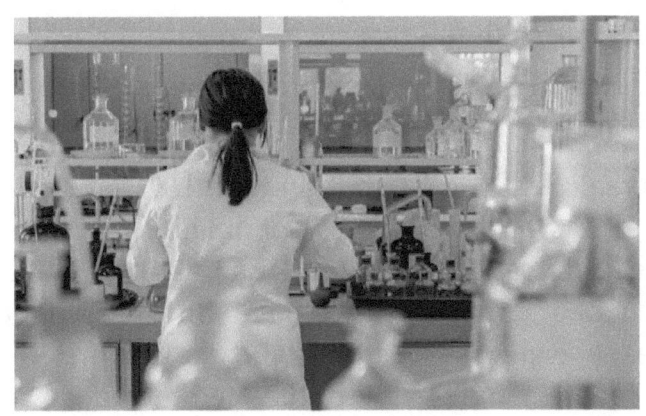

Chapter 3: Mediterranean Diet Recognized by UNESCO

As mentioned at the beginning of the book, the term "Mediterranean diet" was first mentioned by the Americans in the 1960s, most likely in the early years. It became more popular in the 1990s, but only recently, it received the recognition it deserves from UNESCO. Now you are probably thinking what UNESCO has to do with a diet, a meal plan.

As you already know, UNESCO dedicates its activity to preserving the cultural heritage of the world, and as it happens, the Mediterranean diet is considered "pure art" and should be preserved at all costs. This organization has declared that this cookery culture specific to the people living on the shores of the Mediterranean Sea represents a "cultural heritage of humanity."

"This recognition by UNESCO values and emphasizes these, long universally appreciated and approved culinary practices as part of a wider popular culture wherein quality, simplicity and healthfulness of autochthonous (native) food products marry with food folkway practices, with territoriality, biodiversity and with full respect and regard for seasonality. All these attributes co-jointly acquire a determining and characterizing role as a reference point for excellence."[6]

UNESCO realized the contribution that the Mediterranean diet makes to the world's culture and included it as part of its Intangible Cultural Heritage of Humanity on November 17, 2013. Such an organization sees the Mediterranean diet as a set of knowledge, expertise, customs, and skills expressed over the centuries by the people living in the Mediterranean areas, such as Portugal, Spain, Morocco, Italy, Croatia, Greece, and Cyprus "into a nutritional model based on the cultural environment, landscape, crops, preservation, processing, preparation and in particular consumption of food. This model, consisting primarily of olive oil, cereals, fresh and dried fruit, vegetables, a moderate quantity of fish, meat and dairy produce, a variety of condiments and spices, all washed down with wine or teas, has remained constant in time and space. A cultural expression or practice is included in the intangible cultural heritage of humanity list either due to an urgent need to preserve it or due to its representative status."[7]

Although there are many definitions when it comes to this diet, most of the authors and specialists would agree that the Mediterranean diet consists of the following:

[6] Saulle, R. and La Torre, G. (2010). Retrieved from
https://www.researchgate.net/publication/288123570_The_Mediterranea
n_Diet_recognized_by_UNESCO_as_a_cultural_heritage_of_humanity

[7] Europarl.europa.eu. (2014). The Mediterranean diet, part of UNESCO's intangible cultural heritage of humanity. Retrieved from http://www.europarl.europa.eu/doceo/document/E-8-2014-010814_EN.html

- Higher consumption of cereals, fruits, pulses (lentils, beans, etc.) and vegetables

- Medium to high consumption of fish

- Low consumption of saturated fat and meat

- Higher levels of unsaturated fat (especially olive oil)

- Low to medium dairy products intake (yogurt and cheese)

- Moderate red wine consumption

All of the above seem to form a pattern that occurs in many Mediterranean countries. Moreover, if you think of the current times we are living (when most of our food is processed at an industrial level, is extremely calorie-dense, and has little to no nutritional value), this may be the perfect time to promote a healthier alternative to our daily food eating habits.

This may have a downside, though, as excessive advertising of this diet "may fade typical regional identity and membership profiles, tending toward a depersonalization of the authentic eno-gastronomic folkways and customs, and to counteract this, the UNESCO takes sides in defence of genuineness, flavour, food taste and chiefly health promotion in order to promote healthy eating habits, handing over the legitimized sceptre to 'our' peculiar food tradition as well as to our benevolent good nature."[8]

Most of the credit for the UNESCO recognition should be due to the epidemiological and ethnological research conducted for this term. The epidemiological research focuses on human habits, geographical distribution, and diversity while the

---

[8] Saulle, R. and La Torre, G. (2010). Retrieved from https://www.researchgate.net/publication/288123570_The_Mediterranean_Diet_recognized_by_UNESCO_as_a_cultural_heritage_of_humanity

ethnological one is all about the birth of this term, as formulated by the American researcher Ancel Keys. At that time, this researcher also mentioned the protective and beneficial effects of this diet. The epidemiological research proves the positive impact that the Mediterranean diet can have on your health, with implications on myocardial infarction, stroke, cardiovascular and respiratory diseases, cancer, dyslipidemia, hypertension, and diabetes. More details regarding the studies conducted and the effects of this diet on these diseases and conditions can be seen in the previous chapter.

There are organizations that consider obesity as a serious public health issue as it rapidly becomes more of a global epidemic. The main causes of the booming trend of obesity are already known, as it's closely linked with the high consumption of processed food and drinks. The Italian lifestyle, which should have been a Mediterranean one, has become more westernized—meaning, the Italian people consume junk food more than ever, and they are less active as they used to be. Besides all these, the consumption of animal fats and meat is skyrocketing.

The Mediterranean diet should be considered more than a diet. It is a tradition, a culture, and above all, a sustainable and high-quality art. Unfortunately, today only the people living in the rural areas of the Mediterranean basin (and mostly elderly people) still follow this diet. They pay more attention to their health, and they also have access to organic food and are a lot less exposed to processed and junk food.

UNESCO's goal is to promote this dietary plan and lifestyle among younger people. The organization also aims to spread this lifestyle at a European level by conducting different nutritional campaigns and presenting the Mediterranean diet as a cultural heritage for humanity. This organization values the point recently adopted by the Istanbul Declaration of the World Federation of Public Health Associations that "the rights and the healthy traditions and cultures of indigenous people and communities need to be recognized, respected, promoted and protected."[9] Therefore, it does its best to achieve the goals of promoting and protecting the Mediterranean diet and way of life.

Chapter 4: Differences from Other Diets

Let's think about most of the diets known today to man. What do most of them have in common? Some of them propose to eliminate some food types. Others impose meal plans for a limited amount of time. Other diets simply want you to count calories. Others impose a very strict feeding schedule (there are some diets that are known to combine the restriction of standard diets with the practice of intermittent fasting). Only a few of them are actually suggesting a lifestyle, something that you can hold on for the rest of your life. Other diets recommend a meal plan of four different days, each day focusing on one food type. Most of them are found to be too radical, not that easy to follow, and only have results on the short run.

A standard diet focuses on losing weight, not on real health benefits. That's why most people think they go on a diet to lose weight, not to achieve other benefits. Who would think that they go on a diet to improve their cognitive function and to

---

9 Saulle, R. and La Torre, G. (2010). Retrieved from https://www.researchgate.net/publication/288123570 The Mediterranean Diet recognized by UNESCO as a cultural heritage of humanity

make their brain work better?

People nowadays are always stressed about losing more weight in a record amount of time. What they don't realize is that a healthy weight loss can be achieved through working out, and they also have to follow a healthy diet in order to prepare the body for the weight loss process.

The modern-day lifestyle involves too much sedentarism, too much stress, and not too much time for proper meals. Also, we are bombarded by processed and junk food. Most radical diets promise you the impossible. They always advertise that you will be able to lose an incredible amount of pounds (or kilos) in record time; all you have to do is follow a certain plan and renounce eating certain food types. These meal plans are for a very limited amount of time. They may promise to deliver what you are expecting, but in most cases, they are not backed up by scientific research. What they don't mention are the side effects, as many of these diets can be harmful to your body.

Let's say that you want to lose weight by following a meal plan for one week or a month. You will see the obvious results, and you will congratulate yourself for taking that particular diet and for being ambitious enough to stick to it. Sticking to such diets requires you to have a very strong will and ambition. If you switch back to your standard processed-food diet, you will find yourself gaining weight at an even faster pace.

Most of the diets known today are too restrictive—basically determining you to stick just to one or a few food types. Remember, your body needs all the macronutrients (proteins, carbohydrates, fats), as well as minerals and vitamins, in order to function properly. These diets will not cover your basic nutritional needs, so they are not an option for a longer period of time, not even in the short term.

You can find below some of the main features of today's diets:

Nutrient Deprivation

This is common to the meal plans or diets that impose just a few food types, which simply can't cover the basic nutritional needs. Do you think a vegan diet can cover your requirements in terms of nutrients? It simply can't.

Caloric Deprivation

Counting the calories you eat is starting to become an obsession for people on a diet. But when the meal plan imposes a daily calorie consumption of 800–1,000 calories, that's when you will experience hunger.

Too Many Rules

If you want to lose weight using such diets, you need to follow the rules. In many cases, these rules are too strict, so many people on diet plans find themselves quitting the diet relatively quickly.

Restrictions

These restrictions refer not only to the accepted food type or the number of calories consumed. It can also mean the feeding schedule.

Not Scientifically Researched

When it comes to taking a diet plan, most people browse the internet for information, but the information they stumble on might be false. Most diets guarantee that you will lose a certain number of pounds (or kilos) in record time. How many people actually lost that much weight as advertised by the diet? Not all bodies are the same, and people don't have the same metabolism. Such diets may be promoted by people who are specialists in this domain just because they invented a meal plan that had some impressive results on their body. When choosing a diet plan, people should also consider the research studies on this diet. Above all, they need to consult a doctor or a nutritionist to find out whether a specific diet is right for them.

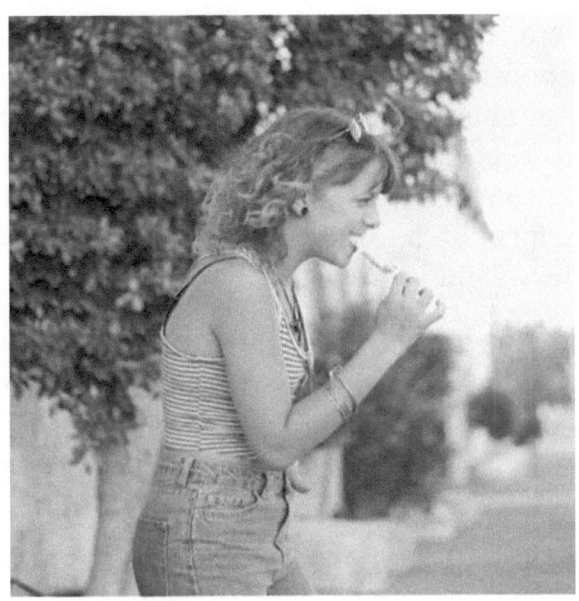

Possible Side Effects

When on a diet, you may lose weight, but to what cost? Is it worth it to damage your health on such a meal plan? That's why you need to have a principle when choosing a diet. That principle should be "Health first." Find out everything about the diet you are about to take, not just the food you need to eat. If you discover some dangerous side effects, you need to stop there and abandon the diet immediately.

These are just a few features of diets today. Most of them mean food-type deprivation (or just calorie), time limitation, strict rules, or feeding schedule. They are all focused on the weight loss process, ignoring the possible side effects. Most people can't stick to diets because they are too harsh; thus, they need to abandon their dream of losing weight extremely fast.

What if there is a diet out there that doesn't involve deprivation, doesn't stress you about losing weight extremely fast, and doesn't harm your health? This book has an answer to this question. The Mediterranean diet is everything other diets are not as it promotes a healthier lifestyle. After all, a healthy body can perform at its best, so it is most likely to be more efficient at the weight loss process.

You don't have to quit eating your favorite meal type unless that food type is processed. This diet allows you to eat almost anything as long as you eat natural and organic. It's really hard to think of a meal plan that has more allowed types of food than the Mediterranean diet.

If you check this diet's food pyramid, you will definitely find your food type in there. By respecting the pyramid, you will understand how often you can eat a certain food type. More details regarding the ingredients of this meal plan and its pyramid can be found in other chapters of this book.

The Mediterranean diet is designed to bring more balance to your life. It is a lifestyle and not just about eating. Guess what the Mediterranean diet pyramid has at its base? It's physical exercise! The diet promotes this kind of activity first on a daily basis.

This kind of diet has a complete LCHF (low-carb, high-fat) meal plan. It means you consume high levels of healthy fats and lower levels of carbs. This diet encourages only moderate consumption of bread or pasta. If you eat them, they should be made out of whole grains with lower carb concentration. This leads to a decent carb level—not as low as the ketogenic diet but still at a very good level.

Moreover, there is no mention of how much food you can eat, so you can forget about nutrient deprivation. The natural food of this meal plan is more nutrient-dense than calorie-dense, and this extends your satiety level for a longer period. This means that you will not experience hunger while being on this diet. Unlike other diets, this one was intensively researched, and the results were just incredible. There are plenty of health benefits (and also mental and physical benefits) backed up with scientific studies. More benefits can be found in a previous chapter.

The Mediterranean diet is an art, as it comprises not only the eating habits of the people from the Mediterranean basin but also their lifestyle, activities, and culture. It's no wonder that UNESCO has chosen this meal plan to be a part of their cultural heritage. It promotes a healthier and stress-free lifestyle. You don't have to worry about weight loss as you will definitely experience it.

Also, the diet sets the right expectations, so it doesn't promise an incredible number of pounds or kilos lost without being able to deliver. The food you eat prepares the body for the weight loss (fat loss) process, making it healthier and increasing its performance. Combined with an active lifestyle with proper physical activity, your body is in optimal condition to lose weight.

Chapter 5: Obesity Is a Worldwide Problem

There are plenty of problems that humanity is facing today, and obesity is one of the most serious ones. This physical condition is the result of several factors:

- Calorie-dense food

- Sedentarism

- Stress and an agitated lifestyle

Most diseases known today are caused by improper alimentation, mostly because of processed food. Finding proper organic and natural food has become a real challenge by most people living in urban areas in the Western world. Just think about it! Obesity was not a phenomenon a few centuries ago. This condition developed a lot in the last decades. Responsible for spreading it is the fast-food restaurants and the supermarkets, which promote mostly processed food.

Processed food is the kind of food that is industrially made based on different kind of ingredients. The problem is that, in most cases, those ingredients are not natural. They are instead chemicals that can be extremely harmful to your body. For the sake of profit, food companies have replaced natural ingredients with different chemicals to fool the consumer (those chemicals can give an interesting flavor to the product that is very close to the natural one). However, these chemicals can't cover the nutritional requirements of your body as natural food would. This is why processed food is only calorie-dense, not nutrient-dense.

Supermarkets are all about buying extremely cheap food

products from manufacturers (in bulk), and in order for these manufacturers to stay in business, they have to lower the cost of production. The most common method is to use chemicals instead of natural ingredients. This is how they can keep profits up and remain in business, although they are literally producing poison.

There is no national or international agency to stand up for the consumer and impose the manufacturing of more natural food. People are aware of what they are consuming (each processed product is properly labeled and shows the nutritional value), but in many cases, they can't afford to buy natural food as it's significantly more expensive. Most of the products on the supermarket's shelves are processed, as the target consumers can afford just this kind of food. Natural food is more perishable, so it has to be consumed fresh. You have to buy it more often, and since it's already more expensive, purchasing it more frequently can leave you with empty pockets.

Most people nowadays have to pay plenty of bills, loans, or mortgages; so the budget for food is significantly decreased. This is how people mostly buy this kind of food. In many Western countries, the middle class is becoming "extinct." People are either getting rich or fall into poverty. Well, guess what kind of food the poor people are eating?

Obesity is more frequent in the lower-income class. Rich people can afford natural food, so they are not that exposed to the effects of processed food. Fast-food restaurants are developing more than ever, and they are very popular as they promote extremely cheap food with little to no nutritional value. They run on processed food, so we can honestly say that they helped a lot with the spread of obesity.

Processing food at an industrial scale also affects the most basic types of food. Chemicals and fertilizers are used for growing crops, vegetables, and fruits. Animals are fed with concentrated food in order to grow at an incredible pace before getting slaughtered for meat. This is how the chemicals used in treating plants or feeding animals end up in our diet.

Most of the food sold in supermarkets or in restaurants is exactly as the ones mentioned above. Finding true organic food is a very difficult challenge, as people living in the urban areas of the Western world don't have access to such food. Why buy fresh fish and cook it yourself when you can already find in supermarkets a breaded and spiced one (prepared to be fried)?

Simple fish fillets are very good, but adding extras to them, such as breading and other condiments, automatically increases the level of carbs. Very high levels of carbs found in processed food and particularly junk food (e.g., burgers, pizza, and French fries) cause obesity.

Carbohydrates have a special compound called glucose, which is basically sugar. Glucose is used by the body to generate energy. Just take a look at the label of any soft drink or fruit juice to see the sugar level in it. It's kind of terrifying, right? Glucose can be burned only through physical activity. This is how energy is generated. However, when there's no physical activity, the glucose that is not used gets stored in your blood, raising the insulin and blood sugar level. Glucose is the default "fuel type" in this case. Processed food doesn't contain only glucose; it also contains high levels of unhealthy fats. Since the body runs on glucose, which is not used entirely, guess what happens with the fat you consume? It gets added to your fat tissue. If you don't work out, you will not be able to burn fat, so it will continue to get stored to your fat tissue. This is how you get obese.

Physical activity can be one of the most important enemies of obesity. Eating processed food will not guarantee excess energy. On the contrary, you will feel more tired and less willing to try any type of physical activity. Since processed food also causes addiction (your body craves for more carbs and glucose from this type of food), you can also say that it causes fatigue, so it encourages sedentarism.

You definitely need more vitality. You need to escape from this vicious circle of continuously having processed food in order to become more active. The more you burn glucose, the more you feel energized. It's the physical activity that generates energy, not eating copious numbers of carbs rich in glucose.

Burning fat should be the ultimate goal of physical activity, whether you are jogging, cycling, swimming, or working out at the gym. Once your body is in the fat-burning mode, the fat tissue is slowly getting replaced by muscle mass. If you ask any fat or obese person, their main goal is to lose weight. Perhaps turning most of their fat tissue into muscle mass is not something they desire, but that can be avoided through a proper diet.

The number of proteins you consume each day can maintain, increase, or decrease your muscles. If you are obese, you probably want to decrease the muscle mass also, but most of all, you want to burn fat. There are studies that showed impressive results from HIIT (high-intensity interval training). This type of training incorporates endurance training with high intensity. Apparently, lifting heavy weights a few times, followed by a short break of just a few seconds, and then repeating the exercise and break a few times can have outstanding results in terms of fat burning. Also, big weights activate the growth hormone, so you will gain bigger muscles. If you are not planning on becoming a massive bodybuilder in a distant future, then cardio exercises and lifting very light weights with many repetitions can be what you are looking for. This will definitely burn your fat, and the growth hormone will not be activated. So if you have a low-protein diet, you will lose muscle mass.

Obesity is also favored by stress and an agitated way of life. The modern-day job involves doing plenty of tasks during a working schedule, and tight deadlines are something very common. People often stay overtime to finish their task, or they don't have the necessary time to have a proper meal or to work out. This agitated and stressful way of life is associated with irregular feeding, and this is definitely something that causes obesity. Not having a fixed schedule for eating and eating very late is often not a healthy habit. Having a consistent meal just before going to bed will not allow your body to burn the calories you just ate. This is a very unhealthy habit that will make you gain weight in no time.

Higher stress levels also mean plenty of snacks. People tend to eat more snacks when they are stressed. Those snacks are simply caloric bombs. They create the illusion of satiety, but this feeling only lasts for a few moments. Most likely, you feel hungry again in an hour (or something like that). Usually, the kinds of snacks that are the most harmful are chips, nachos, or other kinds of processed foods. The body becomes addicted to them, and that is why stressed people eat more often these kinds of snacks than real food.

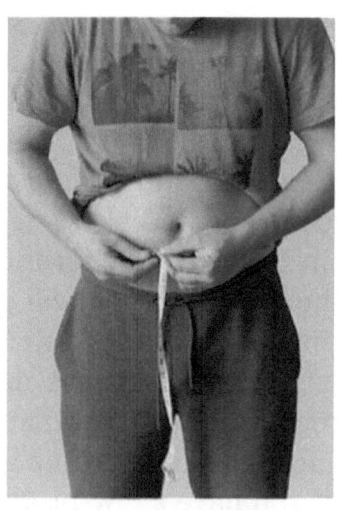

Chapter 6: Ingredients of the Mediterranean Diet

Most diet plans will make you throw out almost everything you have in your refrigerator. It's a shame to waste food just because it doesn't comply anymore with your diet plan. When it comes to the Mediterranean diet, you will be able to keep plenty of food you have in your refrigerator, but you will not be able to keep most processed food. In order to make things easier for you, you have to respect a shopping list for this diet, containing the most important ingredients.

These ingredients are structured into eleven different categories, as seen below:

1. Vegetables

2. Fruits

3. Dairy

4. Meat and poultry

5. Fish and seafood

6. Grains and bread

7. Fats and nuts

8. Beans

9. Pantry items

10. Herbs and spices

11. Greens

The vegetable category can include frozen veggies, such as green beans, peas, or spinach; but you need mostly fresh veggies, such as romaine lettuce, cabbage, spinach, beets, celery leaves, carrots, broccoli, cauliflower, mushrooms, potatoes, peas, garlic, zucchini, okra, green beans, cucumbers, eggplant, onions, peppers, and tomatoes.

The fruits section of your shopping list must include apricots, figs, pears, peaches, cantaloupe, watermelon, cherries, pears, apples, lemons, tangerines, and oranges.

Dairy products can be a very interesting fat source, but milk is not included in here. As nutritious as it may be for a growing body, milk is no longer considered an eligible food type for the Mediterranean diet. The dairy category includes mizithra, graviera, fresh mozzarella, Parmesan, ricotta (or other fresh cheese), feta cheese, Greek yogurt (strained yogurt), and sheep's milk yogurt.

Meat or poultry doesn't represent a very important category in this diet. You are only allowed to eat them twice a week. Still, you have to include them in your diet. You can buy, in this case, chicken (a whole chicken, thighs, or breast), pork, veal, or ground beef. You can get plenty of proteins from eating this kind of food, but the protein intake is still in the required parameters for this diet.

What is a Mediterranean diet without fish or seafood? Although you don't have it every day, it's about the same frequency as poultry or meat. Your shopping list for this diet should not be without calamari, octopus, shrimp, cod, sardines (you can have them canned or fresh), and anchovies (again, you can have them fresh or canned).

People nowadays seem to abuse bread and other types of pastry. This eating habit is not considered healthy, and these food types should only be consumed moderately. Even when they are consumed, it's highly recommended to consume products made out of whole grains. This diet doesn't exclude the consumption of bread and pastries. In fact, you can consume products like couscous, bulgur, egg pasta, rice, pasta, phyllo, pita bread, breadsticks made from whole grains, paximadi (barley rusks), and bread (made from whole grains).

There isn't a Mediterranean diet without healthy fats, such as olive oil. Also, this meal plan emphasizes the consumptions of nuts. You will have to make sure that your shopping list includes sesame seeds, pistachios, pine nuts, walnuts, almonds, tahini, and of course, extra-virgin olive oil.

Eating beans is also included in this meal plan; therefore, you will have to consume fava (yellow split pea), chickpeas, white beans, and lentils.

If you are not sure what pantry items are, in this category, you can find wine (preferably red) honey, balsamic vinegar (or red wine vinegar), capers, sundried tomatoes, olives, tomato paste, and canned tomatoes.

Herbs and spices play a very important role in the Mediterranean diet as this category enhances the flavor of the food you eat. That's why it shouldn't be missing from any cooked meals in this dietary plan. When following this diet, you need to include on your shopping list (if you don't have them already) herbs and spices, such as herbal teas (chamomile, sage, thyme), black pepper and sea salt, cinnamon, cumin, basil, mint, dill, parsley, oregano, and all kind of spices.

The last category is represented by greens, but they still are a very important part of this diet. You can find in here amaranth, beet greens, dandelion, and chicory. It sounds very interesting, right? This is a very impressive shopping list, and since there are plenty of perishable foods on this list, you need to buy fresh frequently. Remember, food waste is something you will have to avoid, especially when it comes to healthy food types, such as the ones included here. Therefore, in order to be sure you will consume each food type and ingredient included in this list, you have to establish a meal plan, a detailed menu for each day of the week.

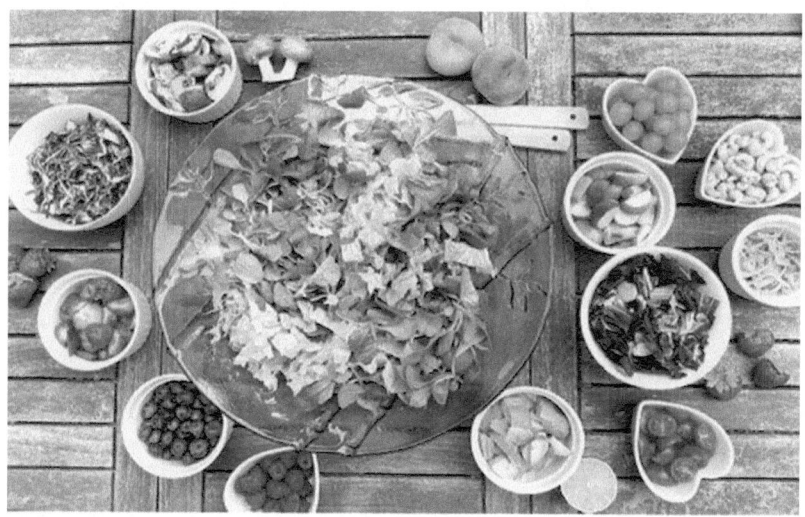

Chapter 7: Breakfast

Many people believe that breakfast is the most important meal of the day as it should provide you with the caloric boost you need to get you started. Breakfast plays an essential role in the Mediterranean diet, which is a dietary plan that includes all the important meals of the day, plus snacks or dessert. This chapter includes some of the most delicious recipes for the first meal of the day.

Potato and Chickpea Hash[10]

A special meal you can have for breakfast is the potato and chickpea hash. This is a meal that can be prepared fast and easy, and it shouldn't take more than 15 minutes to prepare and cook it.

Ingredients

- 4 large egg

- 1 can chickpeas (the chickpeas will have to be rinsed)

- 1 cup chopped zucchini

- ¼ cup extra-virgin olive oil

- ½ teaspoon sea salt

- 1 tablespoon curry powder

- 2 cups chopped baby spinach

- ½ cup chopped onion

- 1 tablespoon ginger (freshly minced)

- 4 cups shredded hash brown potatoes

Directions

1. In a large bowl, combine the potatoes, ginger, onion, spinach, curry powder, and sea salt.

---

[10] McDonell, L. (2016). The Mediterranean diet for beginners: 110 delicious recipes and the complete guide to going Mediterranean, pp. 48–49.

2. In a nonstick skillet set over medium-high heat, heat extra-virgin olive oil and add the potato mixture.

3. Press the mixture into a layer and cook for about 5 minutes without stirring or until golden brown and crispy.

4. Lower heat to medium-low and fold in zucchini and chickpeas, breaking up the mixture until just combined.

5. Stir briefly. Press the mixture back into a layer and make four wells.

6. Break one egg into each indentation.

7. Cook covered for about 5 minutes or until eggs are set.

Mediterranean Pancakes[11]

Who wouldn't love to have pancakes for breakfast? Well, why not have some Mediterranean pancakes? As you may imagine, preparing such a delicious breakfast takes much longer than making an omelet. It should take around 50 minutes, including 30 minutes of preparation time, plus another 20 minutes to cook them. You should be able to get around 16 pancakes by getting this recipe right.

Ingredients

- fresh fruits (berries preferably)
- syrup or other toppings
- 2 tablespoons honey
- 2 cups nonfat Greek yogurt
- 2 large eggs
- 2 tablespoons extra-virgin olive oil
- ¼ teaspoon sea salt
- 1 teaspoon baking soda
- 2 tablespoons flax seeds
- ½ cup flour
- 1 cup old-fashioned oats

---

[11] McDonell, L. (2016). The Mediterranean diet for beginners: 110 delicious recipes and the complete guide to going Mediterranean. Independently Published, pp. 51–52.

Instructions

1. In a blender, combine oats, flour, flax seeds, baking soda, and sea salt. Blend for about 30 seconds.

2. Add extra-virgin olive oil, eggs, yogurt, and honey and continue pulsing until very smooth.

3. Let the mixture stand for at least 20 minutes or until thick.

4. Set a large nonstick skillet over medium heat and brush with extra-virgin olive oil.

5. In batches, ladle the batter by quarter-cupfuls into the skillet.

6. Cook the pancakes for about 2 minutes or until bubbles form and golden brown.

7. Turn them over and cook the other sides for 2 minutes more or until golden brown.

8. Transfer the cooked pancakes to a baking sheet and keep warm in the oven.

9. Serve with favorite toppings.

Breakfast Couscous

Another delicious recipe is the breakfast couscous. This is the kind of meal that can be made fast and easy. In order to prepare 4 portions, you don't need more than 15 minutes—10 minutes for preparation time and 5 minutes for cook time.

Ingredients

- 4 teaspoons melted butter
- ¼ teaspoon sea salt
- ½ cup chopped dried apricots
- ¼ cup dried currants
- 6 teaspoons brown sugar
- 1 cup whole-wheat couscous
- 3 cups semi-skimmed milk (1% fat)
- 1 cinnamon stick

Directions

1. Mix the milk and the cinnamon stick in a saucepan at medium heat but just for 3 minutes (you don't need to boil the milk).

2. Put the pan aside and place in the currants, apricots, sea salt, sugar, and the couscous. Stir them all together until you get the mixture. Let it stand (you need to cover it first) for at least 15 minutes.

3. Get rid of the cinnamon stick and split the couscous into

4 different portions. Place on top of each portion 1 teaspoon of melted butter and ½ teaspoon of brown sugar.

4. The food is now ready, so you can serve it immediately.

Creamy Paninis[12]

Do you like paninis? Then you can have them for breakfast, as you can find the recipe below. In order to prepare 4 portions of paninis, you will only need 15 minutes.

Ingredients

- 7 ounces of sliced, roasted red peppers

- 4 slices provolone cheese

- 1 small zucchini, thinly sliced

- 4 slices bacon

- 4 slices whole-wheat bread

- ½ cup mayonnaise dressing made with olive oil

- ¼ cup freshly chopped basil leaves

- 2 tablespoons oil-cured and finely chopped black olives

Cooking Instructions

1. In a small bowl, combine olives, basil, and ¼ cup of mayonnaise. Evenly spread the mayonnaise mixture on the bread slices and layer 4 slices with bacon, zucchini, provolone, and peppers.

2. Top with the remaining bread slices and spread the

---

[12] McDonell, L. (2016). The Mediterranean diet for beginners: 110 delicious recipes and the complete guide to going Mediterranean. Independent Publisher, p. 46.

remaining ¼ cup of mayonnaise on the outside of the sandwiches. Cook over medium heat for about 4 minutes, turning once until cheese is melted and the sandwiches are golden brown.

Breakfast Stir-Fry

For this recipe, you need around 25 minutes, which includes 5 minutes prep time, plus 20 minutes of cooking. In the end, you will have 4 portions.

Ingredients

- 4 chopped tomatoes
- 2 finely chopped onions
- 2 sliced green peppers
- 1 tablespoon extra-virgin olive oil
- ½ teaspoon sea salt
- 1 egg

Cooking Instructions

1. Use a frying pan to heat the olive oil at medium-high heat.

2. Put the sauté and green pepper for about 2 minutes in the pan.

3. At this point, you need to decrease the heat to medium and continue cooking for about 3 minutes.

4. Put the onion and stir until it gets brown. It should be around 2 minutes.

5. Stir in the salt and tomatoes. Simmer and cover until you have a soft juicy mixture.

6. Beat the egg in a separate bowl and drizzle it over the

mixture. Cook it for 1 minute without stirring.

7. Once this is made, you can serve the dish with black olives, feta cheese, and cucumber slices. Enjoy it!

Zucchini and Tomato Frittata

It takes around 15 minutes to prepare this dish, and once it's done, you should have enough of it for 2 portions.

Ingredients

- 8 crushed eggs
- ¼ teaspoon crushed red pepper
- 1 tablespoon olive oil
- 1 thinly sliced zucchini
- ½ cup halved cherry tomatoes
- 2 ounces mozzarella balls
- ⅓ cup chopped walnuts

Cooking Directions

1. Preheat the skillet. Whisk the eggs with crushed red pepper and sea salt in a medium bowl.

2. Put olive oil in the skillet over medium heat. At the bottom of the skillet, add the zucchini slices for approximately 3 minutes, and then turn them once.

3. Pour the egg mixture but also add the cherry tomatoes over the zucchinis into the skillet. Also, add on top walnuts and mozzarella balls and then cook them all for about 5 minutes.

4. Put aside the skillet for approximately 4 minutes until it is set.

5. Cut into wedges and serve with basil leaves and slices of tomatoes. Also, make sure you pour olive oil.

Mediterranean Breakfast Sandwich

For this food type, you need to allocate yourself around 20 minutes, which include the whole cooking and preparing process. In the end, you will have sandwiches for 4 servings.

Ingredients

- 4 multigrain sandwich thins
- 4 teaspoons olive oil
- 1 tablespoon fresh rosemary
- 4 eggs
- 2 cups baby spinach leaves
- 1 thinly sliced medium tomato
- 4 tablespoons reduced feta cheese
- ⅛ teaspoon kosher salt and black pepper (freshly ground)

Cooking Directions

1. Preheat the oven at 375 °F.

2. Divide the sandwich thins and brush the cut sides using 2 teaspoons of olive oil.

3. On a baking sheet, place the sandwich thins and then let them toast in the oven for approximately 5 minutes until you notice that the edges are light brown and the thins are becoming crisp.

4. Put a large skillet on the stove at medium heat and then

add the remaining olive oil (2 teaspoons). Put some rosemary also, and let it cook.

5. Break eggs into the skillet and let it cook for 1 minute (or until you notice that the whites are set and the yolks are becoming runny).

6. Use a spatula to break the yolks and then flip the eggs to be cooked on one side until it's well done. At this point, put the skillet aside and turn off the heat.

7. You need to place the toasted sandwich thins into 4 different plates and then add some tomato slices, 1 egg, and a teaspoon of feta cheese.

8. Don't forget to sprinkle some olive oil again and enjoy.

Breakfast Burrito[13]

This meal doesn't sound Mediterranean at all, but you can cook it in such a style. It takes around 20 minutes to get 6 portions.

Ingredients

- 6 tortillas

- 9 eggs

- 2 cups of baby spinach

- 3 tablespoons of black olives

- 3 tablespoons of chopped sun-dried tomatoes

- ½ cup feta cheese

- salsa for garnish

- ¾ cup of canned refried beans

Cooking Directions

1. Use nonstick spray to spray a medium pan and then place over medium heat. Scramble eggs and toss for about 5 minutes.

2. Add spinach, sun-dried tomatoes, and black olives. Continue to stir until no longer wet. Add feta cheese and then cover. Cook until the cheese is melted.

---

[13] Volia, I. (n.d.). Mediterranean diet for beginners: With over 120 best healthy food recipes, meal plan to lose weight. Independently Published, p. 45.

3. Add 2 tablespoons of the refried beans on each tortilla and then top with the egg mixture. Divide equally between all the burritos and then wrap.

4. Grill the burritos in a frying pan until lightly browned and then serve hot with salsa and fruit.

Breakfast Buns[14]

This meal is among the most delicious ones you can have for breakfast. It should take around 50 minutes to prepare 4 portions, but it's totally worth cooking it.

Ingredients

- 3 tablespoons of butter
- ½ cup fresh shiitake mushrooms
- 2 spinaches
- 6 fresh sage leaves
- 1 cup baby spinach
- 11 ounces thin pizza crust
- 1½ cups shredded cheddar cheese
- ⅛ teaspoon black pepper

These breakfast buns require some baking in the oven. It may not be the simplest meal to cook, but if you follow the instructions below, you should be able to get some delicious buns.

Cooking Instructions

1. Preheat the oven at 400 °F and place some parchment paper on a baking tray.

---

[14] Volia, I. (n.d.). Mediterranean diet for beginners: With over 120 best healthy food recipes, meal plan to lose weight. Independently Published, pp. 49–51.

2. Put a nonstick skillet at medium heat and then add sausage, mushrooms, and butter. Cook for approximately 4 minutes, stirring until you notice the sausage is properly heated and the mushrooms are tender. Once this is done, place the skillet aside.

3. Beat some eggs in a medium-sized bowl and add some salt and pepper. Whisk them all together until they are properly beaten. In the same skillet, put some butter and leave it to cook over medium heat.

4. Put the egg mixture in the skillet and cook for approximately 3 minutes. Make sure you stir it frequently until the mixture is moist and firm. Add the cheese, continue to stir, and then place the skillet aside. Let it cool for about 10 minutes.

5. On a cutting board, sprinkle some flour. Put the pizza dough on it and make sure you squeeze it into a 14×10-inch rectangle.

6. Make sure you add evenly the sausage, cheese, and eggs mixture and press down slightly. Sprinkle some spinach over the mixture evenly.

7. Pat the sides of the dough to retain a length of approximately 10 inches and then roll it tightly.

8. Pinch the edges to seal. Reshape the buns as you press the tops slowly down. Bake in the oven for about 15 minutes or until golden.

9. Place a skillet over medium heat and then melt about 1 tablespoon of butter. Add sage leaves and then cook for about 2 minutes as you turn frequently until crisp.

10. Remove sage to a paper towel and then crumble.

Reserve the butter in a skillet. Remove the buns from the oven and then brush the sides with the butter that you have reserved. Bake for a minute longer.

11. Sprinkle each of the buns with the crumbled sage leaves and then serve them warm.

Bananas Foster French Toast

Everybody loves French toast, so we can only assume that you will adore this recipe. In order to prepare 4 portions of this meal, you only need around 30 minutes. You will have to prepare a banana sauce and the French toast itself.

Ingredients

For the banana sauce:

- 4 ounces unsalted butter
- ½ cup brown sugar
- 2 tablespoons water
- 4 bananas, peeled and cut

For the French toast:

- 3 whole eggs
- 3 egg yolks
- ½ cup whole milk
- ¼ cup whipping cream
- 6 slices challah bread
- 3 tablespoons unsalted butter
- whipped cream

Instructions

1. Melt some butter in a skillet over medium heat and then add some brown sugar. Whisk until it melts and gets completely mixed with butter. Add some water and make sure you whisk it until the mixture gets smooth. Place aside the skillet and cover it.

2. Whisk the eggs into a separate bowl. Add some cream, milk, and vanilla. Dip the bread slices into the mixture. Make sure you turn them around until they are all soaked and completely moistened.

3. Put a frying pan over medium heat and melt a teaspoon of butter in it. Place the soaked bread in the pan and cook it until it gets golden brown on both sides (you need to turn it over also). It should take around 3 minutes to get the golden brown color on them. Add extra butter for each of the batches.

4. Once the French toast is made, set aside the frying pan. Add bananas to your sauce and cook it until you have the bananas tender. It should take around 3 minutes.

5. Place the French toast on plates and cover them with whipped cream and banana sauce. Enjoy!

Healthy Breakfast Casserole

How long would you spend to cook a healthy breakfast? Do you think it's worth spending an hour on such a meal? If you think it's totally worth it, then you need to check the recipe below. You definitely will not regret it. The healthy breakfast casserole should take you around 60 minutes to fully cook it—out of which 10 minutes is prep time and the remaining 50 minutes is cooking time. If you follow the recipe below, you should end up with 6 portions of this delicious meal.

Ingredients

- 2 tablespoons extra virgin olive oil

- ½ onion (diced)

- 2 diced medium-sized yellow potatoes

- 1 pound of sliced zucchini

- 3 diced portobello mushrooms caps

- 150 grams torn fresh spinach

- 200 grams ricotta

- 2 cups egg whites

- 12 sliced grape tomatoes, each one cut in 3

- roasted and peeled red pepper (3 of them sliced)

- 2 sourdough rolls

- 100 grams grated mozzarella cheese

- 4 tablespoons grated Pecorino Romano cheese

Instructions

1. Turn on the oven and preheat it at 400 °F.

2. On a baking tray, mix potato, onion, and olive oil and then let it roast for at least 15 minutes.

3. In a separate bowl, drizzle zucchini with ½ tablespoon of olive oil. Make sure the zucchini coats well and then place it in the baking tray.

4. Place all the veggies in the oven and then make sure you roast them for 40 minutes or until they have a golden color.

5. In a frying pan, place sautéed mushroom and ½ tablespoon of olive oil. Cook them for approximately 4 minutes.

6. Take the pan aside and also take the mushrooms from it.

7. In the frying pan, place some sautéed chopped spinach and the remaining olive oil. Cook until it's tender.

8. Mix the ricotta and egg whites in a mixing bowl, then set aside.

9. Mix all the veggies, including peppers and grape tomatoes, with the sourdough rolls and squeeze them all into a 9×13-inch baking tray. Put on top the ricotta mixture and sprinkle some mozzarella and pecorino cheese.

10. Place the baking tray in the oven and leave it to bake for approximately 40 minutes. Once it's done, take it out of the oven and let it cool.

11. Cut it into 6 portions and serve.

Lemon Scones

This recipe is less demanding than the previous one, and it's also a lot quicker and easier to cook. You need to allocate around 30 minutes for this meal—prep time is 15 minutes while cooking time is also 15 minutes. Also, by following the recipe, you should end up with 12 portions.

Ingredients

- 1 cup powdered sugar
- 1–2 teaspoon freshly squeezed lemon juice
- zest from 1 lemon
- ¾ cup reduced-fat buttermilk
- ½ teaspoon sea salt
- 2 tablespoons sugar
- ½ teaspoon baking soda
- 2¼ cups flour

Cooking Instructions

1. Turn on the oven and preheat it at 400 °F.

2. Blend sugar, salt, baking soda, and 2 cups of flour in a food processor, then add lemon zest and buttermilk and continue mixing.

3. On a clean surface, sprinkle the remaining flour and then turn out the dough. Make sure you knead the dough at least 6 times and shape it into a ball.

4. Fatten the dough using a rolling pin until you have a half-inch thick circle.

5. Cut the dough into 4 equal wedges. Each wedge has to be cut into 3 different wedges.

6. Put the scones into a baking tray and then let it bake in the preheated oven for about 15 minutes until they are golden brown.

7. Prepare a thin frosting into a small bowl by mixing powdered sugar with lemon juice.

8. Take the scones out of the oven and sprinkle the frosting while they are still hot.

9. Serve immediately.

Egg and Sausage Breakfast Casserole

This type of meal is more demanding as it takes a long time to prepare it, so you probably want to cook it during weekend mornings. You need to have around 1 hour and 25 minutes to spare—out of which 20 minutes is the prep time and the remaining 1 hour and 5 minutes is for cooking. Still, you will end up with 12 portions, so this should give you extra motivation. You will have to prepare the crust and the casserole separately.

Ingredients

For the crust:

- ¾ teaspoons ground pepper
- ¾ teaspoon salt
- 3 tablespoons olive oil
- 2 pounds shredded and peeled russet potatoes

For the casserole:

- 12 ounces chopped turkey sausage
- 4 green onions (thinly sliced)
- ¼ cup diced bell pepper
- ⅓ cup skimmed milk
- 6 large eggs
- 4 egg whites
- ¾ cup shredded cheddar cheese
- 16 ounces low-fat cottage cheese

Cooking Instructions

The crust:

1. Grease a baking tray of 9×13-inch with 1 tablespoon of olive oil while you leave the oven to preheat at 425 °F.

2. Make sure you squeeze the moisture from the potatoes. You can use a paper or kitchen towel.

3. Mix together in a bowl the potatoes, salt, pepper, and the leftover olive oil. Make sure the potatoes are properly coated.

4. Place the mixture into the baking tray. Make sure it's spread equally and leave it to bake for around 20 minutes (or until you notice the potatoes are golden brown on the edges).

The casserole:

1. Lower the oven heat to 375 °F.

2. Use a large skillet to fry the turkey sausage for 2 minutes at medium-high heat or until it's cooked through.

3. Add in the skillet the red bell pepper and green onions and let it cook for 2 minutes or until you notice the red bell pepper is tender.

4. In a separate bowl, mix the cheeses, egg whites, eggs, and skimmed milk. Whisk them all together.

5. Put them all in the large skillet and stir them together. Pour everything over the crust and then put it to bake for 50 minutes. Once it's done, let it cool and then slice it into 12 different portions. Enjoy!

Chapter 8: Lunch

The Mediterranean diet is all about enjoying your meals and taking the time to eat. That's why you will never have a 10-minute lunch when on this diet. Eating together and socializing are also aspects of this meal plan. It's quite the opposite of fast food—not only because the meal plan is a lot healthier but also because it takes longer than this type of food. This chapter will provide you with ideas for nutritious and healthy meals that can be enjoyed at lunchtime.

Pasta with Tomato Sauce and Mushrooms

Although it's part of the Italian cuisine, pasta is not necessarily a part of the Mediterranean diet, as it usually has high levels of carbs. However, there are special kinds of pasta that can be included in such a meal plan. A very interesting meal is the pasta with tomato sauce and mushrooms, a meat type that is done very quickly (it shouldn't take more than 20 minutes to cook this).

Ingredients

- ¼ cup olive oil

- 2 cups chopped Cremini mushrooms

- 1 chopped green bell pepper

- black pepper and sea salt (use to taste)

- ½ cup chopped Spanish onion

- 3 minced garlic cloves

- 6 coriander seeds

- 2 tablespoons chopped fresh parsley

- 1 teaspoon chopped fresh rosemary

- 1 star anise

- 1 tablespoon tomatoes paste

- 2 chopped ripe tomatoes

- 1 pack spiral pasta

- ⅓ cup crumbled feta cheese

Instructions

1. Pour olive oil in a saucepan and heat it at medium-high flame. Then add the bell pepper, Spanish onion, sautéed mushrooms, and garlic until they are fragrant and tender.

2. Add the tomato paste, star anise, coriander seeds, black peppers, parsley, rosemary, salt, and tomatoes, and then stir them all together. Lower the flame to medium-low and continue to cook the sauce until it's ready.

3. Boil the water and cook the pasta according to the instructions on the pack. Drain the water and then add the sauce over the pasta and stir gently to mix. Use crumbled feta to garnish and to serve warm. Enjoy!

Spanish Macarrones with Chicken

Sticking to pasta, here's another delicious recipe that can fit perfectly in your meal plan. The Spanish macarrones with chicken is done in just 35 minutes, and if you follow the recipe, you should easily end up with 4 portions.

Ingredients

- ½ teaspoon salt

- 1 pack whole-wheat macaroni

- 2 teaspoons olive oil

- 1 thinly sliced shallot

- 2 chopped Spanish pimientos

- ½ teaspoon dried sage

- 1 teaspoon dried rosemary

- 1 bay laurel

- 1 pound boneless and skinless chicken thighs, chopped into bite-sized pieces

- 2 puréed ripe tomatoes

- 1 tablespoon tomato paste

- 8 ounces kale leaves chopped and thawed (it can also be frozen)

- ½ cup creamy yogurt

- ½ cup shredded Herreno cheese

Instructions

1. Boil water in a large pot and then add ½ teaspoon of salt and the macaroni. Stir occasionally.

2. Cook the macaroni 2 minutes less than indicated on the package and keep 1 cup of cooking water.

3. In a nonstick pan, heat 1 teaspoon of olive oil at medium heat. When it's hot, just add the bay laurel, rosemary, sage, Spanish pimientos, and the shallot. Cook until the shallot is tender and the herbs are fragrant.

4. Heat the remaining olive oil. Sear the chicken for 3 to 4 minutes and continue stirring.

5. Add the shallot mixture and the chicken to the bowl with macaroni. At this point, you need to stir the kale, tomato paste, and tomato purée.

6. Stir to mix and then take the mixture into a lightly greased baking tray. In a separate bowl, mix the Herreno cheese with the creamy yogurt.

7. Add the cheese mixture on the top of the casserole and then cover the whole thing with a foil. Bake it in a preheated oven at 390 °F for just 15 minutes (until it gets bubbly). Take the foil away and continue to bake for 10–12 minutes. Let it cool and then serve it!

Barley Pilaf with a Twist[15]

This is a healthy dish recommended for this meal plan that can be ready in about 50 minutes. Below you can find the recipe for 6 portions.

Ingredients

- 1 tablespoon olive oil

- ½ cup sliced scallions

- 1 minced garlic clove

- 1 bay leaf

- 1 teaspoon basil

- ½ teaspoon oregano

- ½ teaspoon sage

- 2 cups pearled barley

- 4 cups of water

- 1 vine-ripe chopped tomato

- 4 tablespoons tomato purée

- 16 ounces canned green peas (drained and rinsed)

- 4 cups kale

---

[15] Thornton, A. (2019). Mediterranean diet cookbook for beginners: Easy and healthy Mediterranean recipes for weight loss. Independently Published, p. 105.

- ½ cup hummus

- 2 tablespoons chopped fresh parsley

- 2 tablespoons chopped fresh chives

- ground black pepper and sea salt (to taste)

Directions

1. Heat the olive oil in a large-sized pot over medium heat; now, sauté the scallions until tender and fragrant.

2. Then add the garlic and herbs to the pot and cook for a further 40 seconds or until fragrant.

3. Then bring the barley, water, tomato, and tomato purée to a rapid boil. Immediately reduce the temperature to simmer. Cook for another 40 minutes.

4. Turn off the heat. Add the canned peas, kale, salt, and black pepper to the pot. Cover and allow it to sit in the residual heat for 5 to 6 minutes. Top each serving with hummus, fresh parsley, and chives. Enjoy!

Moroccan Chicken with Aromatic Couscous

Chicken with couscous sounds like a very delicious combination, but this recipe will definitely convince you to try it. You only need 35 minutes to fully cook this meal, and the ingredients are for 6 portions.

Ingredients

For the Moroccan chicken with aromatic couscous:

- 4 tablespoons olive oil

- 1 pound chicken breast, cut into bite-sized chunks

- 2 cloves of minced garlic

- 1 cup chopped shallots

- 1 bay leaf

- 1 teaspoon dried sage

- 1 teaspoon dried basil

- 2 cups homemade vegetable broth

- 2 tablespoons tomato paste

- 1½ cups tomato purée

- black pepper and sea salt (to taste)

For the cinnamon couscous:

- 2 cups Moroccan couscous (kuskus)

- ½ teaspoon salt

- ¼ teaspoon ground cloves

- ½ teaspoon ground coriander

- ½ teaspoon ground cardamom

- 2 cups hot vegetable broth

- 1 tablespoon coconut oil

- grated zest from one orange

Cooking Instructions

1. Heat some olive oil (2 tablespoons) in a Dutch oven at moderate heat. Sear the chicken breast for approximately 6 minutes and make sure you stir periodically for even cooking.

2. In another pot, heat the remaining olive oil and then place the shallots and garlic for around 4–5 minutes until they get tender and aromatic.

3. Put the herbs and then cook for another minute, then put the vegetable broth into the Dutch oven.

4. Raise the temperature and add the tomato purée and paste. You will have to boil the mixture for 4–5 minutes.

5. Lower the temperature after stirring the chicken and cook for 10 to 12 minutes.

6. In a heatproof bowl, place the couscous, vegetable broth, cardamom, coriander, cloves, and salt. Cover the whole thing and leave it to cool for 10 minutes until the couscous is tender.

7. Using a fork stir the couscous and add the orange zest and coconut oil. Divide the whole meal into 6 different portions.

8. Add the chicken stew on top and serve immediately.

Asiago Cheese and Kale Frittata[16]

This meal can be prepared very easy and fast as it takes only 20 minutes to fully cook it.

Ingredients

- 2 tablespoons olive oil
- 1 chopped onion
- 1 teaspoon Italian seasoning mix
- ½ teaspoon red pepper flakes
- ½ teaspoon Spanish paprika
- 1 teaspoon dried parsley flakes
- 2 minced garlic cloves
- 8 eggs
- 6 ounces kale (torn into small pieces)
- 6 ounces shredded Asiago cheese

Directions

1. Start by preheating your oven to 390 °F.

2. Heat the olive oil in an oven-safe skillet over medium heat. Once hot, sauté the onion until tender and fragrant

---

[16] Thornton, A. (2019). Mediterranean diet cookbook for beginners: Easy and healthy Mediterranean recipes for weight loss. Independently Published, p. 102.

or about 4 minutes. Add the seasonings and garlic and continue cooking an additional 30 seconds to 1 minute or until they are aromatic.

3. Next, mix the eggs and double cream until well combined. Add the kale and mix again. Pour the mixture over the sautéed vegetable in the skillet. Lastly, scatter the Asiago cheese over your frittata.

4. Bake in the preheated oven around 9 minutes or until the eggs begin to set.

5. Place on a cooling rack for 5 to 6 minutes before slicing and serving. Bon appétit!

Authentic Tortilla Española con Chorizo

Ingredients

- ½ cup olive oil

- 2 ounces chorizo sausage (cut into bite-sized chunks)

- 1 pound peeled and sliced Yukon Gold potatoes

- ½ purple onion (thinly sliced)

- chili pepper flakes and salt (to taste)

- 1 bell pepper (roasted, peeled, and sliced)

- 8 eggs

- ½ teaspoon Spanish paprika

Cooking Instructions

1. Heat the olive oil in an oven-proof pan at medium-low heat. Add the potatoes and the chorizo sausage and cook them for approximately 9 minutes, turning them on the other side also.

2. Add the chili pepper flakes, onions, salt, and bell pepper to the pan and then stir.

3. Continue to cook until the onions are translucent and the potatoes are tender. Reserve.

4. Whisk the eggs and the Spanish paprika into a separate bowl and then gently pour it over the potato mixture. Place the whole thing back in the oven-proof pan.

5. Cook over moderate heat until you notice the tortilla

start to set. It should take around 8 to 10 minutes. Flip it over on the other side and then cook for another 4 minutes.

6. Place the tortilla into a serving platter and then serve immediately.

Braised Chicken with Olives

This one is a more demanding type of meal, but it is definitely worth spending 1 hour and 50 minutes to cook. It should take around 20 minutes to prepare the ingredients and another hour and a half for cooking. By following the recipe, you can prepare 4 portions of this meal.

Ingredients

- 1 tablespoon extra-virgin olive oil
- 4 chicken legs (skinned and cut into thighs and drumsticks)
- 1 cup chicken broth
- 1 cup dry white wine
- 4 sprigs thyme
- 2 tablespoons chopped fresh ginger
- 2 minced garlic cloves
- 3 diced carrots
- 1 medium diced yellow onion
- 3¾ cups chickpeas (rinsed and drained)
- ½ cup green olives (roughly chopped and pitted)
- ⅓ cup raisins
- 1 cup water

Cooking Instructions

1. Turn on the oven and let it heat at 350 °F.

2. Heat the extra-virgin olive oil in a large oven-proof pan at medium flame.

3. Place each chicken piece into the pan to fry for about 5 minutes on each side until it is crisp and brown on both sides.

4. Put the cooked chicken to a place and set aside.

5. Decrease the heat to medium-low and add ginger, carrots, onion, and garlic to the pan. Let them cook (you need to stir often) for approximately 5 minutes until you see the onion tender and translucent.

6. Put into the pan water, wine, and chicken broth, and let the mixture to boil gently.

7. Place the chicken back in the pot and stir in thyme.

8. Boil the whole thing and then cover.

9. Transfer the pan into the oven and let it braise for 45 minutes.

10. Take out the pan from the oven and then stir in raisins, olives, and chickpeas.

11. Place back the pan into the oven and then leave to braise for another 20 minutes.

12. Take the pan out of the oven and dispose of the thyme. Serve immediately.

Chicken with Lemon, Olives, and Mustard Greens

This is the kind of delicious meal you can cook in about 40 minutes. It takes 10 minutes to prepare the ingredients and 30 minutes to cook. The end result will be 6 portions of pure art.

Ingredients

- 2 tablespoons extra-virgin olive oil

- 6 skinless chicken breast, cut in half crosswise

- ½ cup Kalamata olives

- 1 tablespoon freshly squeezed lemon juice

- 1½ pounds mustard greens, chopped coarsely and with stalks removed

- 1 cup dry white wine

- 4 minced garlic cloves

- 1 medium red onion, thinly sliced

- ground pepper

- salt

- lemon wedges (for serving)

Instructions

1. Heat 1 tablespoon of extra-virgin olive oil in a large pan at medium-high heat.

2. Spice the chicken with sea salt and pepper and then

place half of it into the pan. Cook it for around 8 minutes or until it gets brown on all sides.

3. Place the cooked chicken on a plate and repeat the procedure with the remaining oil and chicken.

4. Lower the heat to medium and add onion and garlic. Cook and stir until it gets tender. It should be around 6 minutes.

5. Add back the chicken (with its natural juice) with the wine and boil.

6. Lower the heat again. Cover the whole thing and cook it for about 5 minutes.

7. Add the greens on top and sprinkle some pepper and sea salt.

8. Cover them again and cook for another 5 minutes until the chicken is opaque and the greens are wilted.

9. Take the pan aside and stir lemon juice and olive.

10. Serve the meal with lemon wedges and accumulated pan juices.

Mediterranean Flounder[17]

There shouldn't be any Mediterranean diet without fish, so below you can find a few recipes on how to cook fish for this meal plan. The Mediterranean flounder is the perfect example. It needs only 40 minutes to fully cook it (10 minutes to prepare the ingredients and 30 minutes to cook it). The end result should be a delicious meal for 4 persons.

Ingredients

- 5 Roma tomatoes

- 2 tablespoons extra-virgin olive oil

- ½ onion, chopped

- 1 pinch Italian seasoning

- 1 pound flounder/halibut/tilapia

- 4 tablespoons capers

- 24 Kalamata olives (chopped and pitted)

- 1 teaspoon freshly squeezed lemon juice

- ¼ cup white wine

- 6 leaves chopped fresh basil

- 3 tablespoons Parmesan cheese

---

[17] McDonell, L. (2016). The Mediterranean diet for beginners: 110 delicious recipes and the complete guide to going Mediterranean. Independently Published, p. 186.

Directions

1. Preheat your oven to 425 °F.

2. Plunge the tomatoes into boiling water and immediately transfer them into a bowl of ice water. Peel the skins and chop them.

3. Add extra-virgin olive oil to a skillet set over medium heat and sauté onions until translucent.

4. Stir in garlic, Italian seasoning, and tomatoes and cook until tomatoes are tender.

5. Stir in wine, lemon juice, capers, olives, and half of the basil.

6. Lower heat and stir in Parmesan cheese. Cook for about 15 minutes or until the mixture is bubbly and hot.

7. Place fish in a baking dish and cover with the sauce. Bake in the preheated oven for about 20 minutes or until fish is cooked through.

Grilled Salmon

Salmon is probably the best kind of fish you can have on this diet as it has high fat concentration. Grilled salmon is very easy and fast to prepare. It takes around 23 minutes, with a prep time of 15 minutes and cooking time of 8 minutes. This recipe makes 4 serving portions.

Ingredients

- 2 tablespoons freshly squeezed lemon juice
- 1 tablespoon minced garlic
- 1 tablespoon chopped fresh parsley
- 4 tablespoons chopped fresh basil
- 4 fillets salmon
- extra-virgin oil
- cracked black pepper and sea salt (to taste)
- 4 chopped green olives
- 4 thin slices lemon

Cooking Instructions

1. Coat lightly a grill rack using olive oil and cooking spray and place the grill 4 inches from the heat. Make sure you heat the grill to medium-high.

2. In a small bowl, mix the basil, parsley, minced garlic, and lemon juice.

3. Use olive oil to coat the salmon, and season it with black

pepper and sea salt.

4. Put garlic mixture on top of each salmon fillet and place them on the heated grill.

5. Grill at high heat for 4 minutes until the edges are becoming white. Flip over and place the fish on an aluminum foil.

6. Lower the heat and continue grilling for another 4 minutes.

7. Placed the grilled salmon to plates and garnish it with green olives and lemon slices.

8. Serve immediately.

London Broil with Bourbon-Sautéed Mushrooms

Ingredients

- ½ teaspoon extra-virgin olive oil

- ½ cup minced shallot

- ¾ pounds halved crimini mushrooms

- 6 tablespoons nonfat beef stock

- 3 tablespoons bourbon

- ½ tablespoon unsalted butter

- 1 tablespoon pure maple syrup

- black pepper (to taste)

- 1 pound lean London broil

- ⅛ teaspoon sea salt

Cooking Instructions

1. Turn on the oven and let it heat at 400 °F.

2. Place a nonstick pan in the oven for approximately 10 minutes.

3. Take it out and pour extra-virgin olive oil. Make sure you coat the pan.

4. Stir in mushrooms and shallots until well mixed. Put it back in the oven and leave it to roast for 15 minutes

using a wooden spatula to stir.

5. Stir in pepper, butter, maple syrup, bourbon, and beef stock. Put back the pan in the oven. Leave it to cook for 10 minutes or until the liquid decreases to half.

6. Take the pan out of the oven and put aside.

7. Put another nonstick pan in the oven and let it heat for approximately 10 minutes.

8. In the meantime, sprinkle ground pepper and salt on the steak and put it in the hot pan.

9. Let it roast in the oven for approximately 14 minutes, turning it once.

10. Take the meat out of the oven and place the mushrooms instead to warm.

11. Put the steak on a cutting board and let it cool for about 5 minutes.

12. Cut the beef into thin slices and add the sautéed mushrooms to serve.

Lemony Pork with Lentils

Ingredients

- 2 tablespoons extra-virgin olive oil
- 4 pork chops (or 4 ounces)
- 2 tablespoons fresh lemon juice
- 1 teaspoon lemon zest
- 1 garlic clove
- 2 tablespoons fresh rosemary
- 1 tablespoon parsley
- 1 tablespoon pure maple syrup
- 6 cups water
- ½ cup green lentils
- 1 shallot
- 1 rib celery
- ½ cup dry sherry
- 1 teaspoon sea salt
- 1 teaspoon unsalted butter
- ¼ teaspoon red pepper flakes

Directions

1. In a zipper bag, mix the extra-virgin olive oil, maple syrup, parsley, rosemary, garlic clove, lemon zest, lemon juice, and pork chops. Refrigerate the mixture for at least 8 hours.

2. Put the green lentils and 3 cups of water in a pan at medium heat and cook for approximately 20 minutes or until you notice the lentils to be tender. Drain and rinse.

3. Turn on the oven and leave it at 350 °F.

4. Heat a nonstick pan at medium-high heat and then add the marinade. Fry the pork for about 2 minutes per side and put the pan in the oven.

5. In the meantime, in a second saucepan, heat 1 teaspoon of extra-virgin olive oil at medium-high heat. Add celery, red pepper flakes, and shallot and lower the heat to medium. Let it cook for around 4 minutes or until it's tender. Also, you have to stir in the lentils until they are properly warmed.

6. Add sea salt and sherry and cook for approximately 2 minutes or until liquid is decreased to half. Stir in the butter until it melts completely.

7. Split the lentil mixture among four plates and add to each serving one pork chop from the first pan.

8. Take it out and get rid of the garlic from marinade in the first pan and sprinkle sherry in the pan. Increase the heat and add sea salt. Let it cook until the liquid is decreased by half.

9. Pour the sauce evenly over each portion and serve.

Healthy Beef and Broccoli

Ingredients

- 8 milliliters vegetable oil
- 100 grams thinly sliced flank steak
- grams cornstarch
- 90 grams broccoli florets
- 60 milliliters water
- 1 green onion, thinly sliced
- ½ shallot, finely chopped
- 1 minced garlic clove
- 1 gram red pepper flakes, crushed
- 1 gram minced fresh ginger
- 5 milliliter honey
- 20 milliliter soy sauce

Cooking Instructions

1. Pour some oil in a pan at medium heat.
2. Stir in beef and cook for approximately 8 minutes or until it is browned.
3. Take the beef out of the pan and put aside.
4. Add garlic, shallot, and green onions in the same pan.

Cook for about 1 minute but don't forget to stir.

5. Put in the broccoli and cook for approximately 5 minutes.

6. In a bowl, mix water with cornstarch until it is properly blended.

7. Use another bowl to mix soy sauce, honey, ginger, and red pepper flakes, then stir them in the cornstarch mixture until it is properly blended.

8. Put the sauce into the pan and cook for approximately 5 minutes until it gets thick.

9. Place the beef and cook for around 3 minutes.

10. Serve with brown rice.

Chapter 9: Snacks

Avocado Chips[18]

Total time: 30 minutes

Number of servings: 4

Ingredients

- 1 large ripe avocado
- ¾ cup freshly grated parmesan
- 1 teaspoon lemon juice
- ½ teaspoon garlic powder
- kosher salt
- ½ teaspoon Italian seasoning
- freshly ground black pepper

Instructions

1. Get the oven preheated to 325 °F and then line the baking dish with parchment paper.

2. In a bowl, mash the avocado and then stir in Parmesan,

---

[18] Volia, I. (n.d.). Mediterranean diet for beginners: With over 120 best healthy food recipes, meal plan to lose weight. Independently Published, p. 134

lemon juice, garlic powder, salt, pepper, and Italian seasoning.

3. Place scoops of the mixture on the baking sheet and leave a space of 3 inches apart between each scoop.

4. Place in the oven and bake until crisp and golden or for 15 minutes.

5. Remove from the oven and then allow to cool.

6. Serve while at room temperature.

Sweet-and-Spicy Meatballs[19]

Total time: 30 minutes

Number of servings: 6

Ingredients

- 16 ounce cooked meatballs
- ½ tablespoon crushed red pepper
- ½ teaspoon cayenne pepper
- 12 ounces grape jelly
- 1 cup water
- chopped green onions (to be used for garnish)

Instructions

1. Add the cooked meatballs into the pot. In a bowl, mix the grape jelly, chili sauce, spices, and water and then combine.

2. Pour the mixture into the pot and stir. Cover and lock the lid.

3. Set to cook on high pressure for 10 minutes and then quickly release pressure once ready.

4. Let the meatballs cool. After that, serve and garnish with green onions.

---

[19] Volia, I. (n.d.). Mediterranean diet for beginners: With over 120 best healthy food recipes, meal plan to lose weight. Independently Published, p. 122.

Whipped Coconut Cream with Berries

Total time: 15 minutes

Number of serving: 1

Ingredients

- 1 can unsweetened full-fat coconut milk

- berries of choice

- dark chocolate (optional)

Instructions

1. Cool the coconut milk for about 12 hours. Leave it overnight in the refrigerator.

2. Take out the thick part and make sure you leave the water.

3. Use a mixer to whip it for about 3 minutes.

4. Blend the berries.

5. Use chocolate shavings to top the cream.

Toasted Spicy Almonds

Total time: 1 hour 10 minutes

Number of servings: 6

Ingredients

- 4 cups almonds

- 2 tablespoons butter

- 1 teaspoon ground cinnamon

- 1 tablespoon vanilla extract

- 2 egg whites

- 1 teaspoon salt

Instructions

1. Preheat the oven at 450 °F.

2. Add into a bowl all the ingredient except the almonds and stir until everything is properly mixed.

3. Next, add the almonds to the mixture and mix until well coated.

4. Place the mixture into a baking tray. Bake it for approximately 10 minutes and stir occasionally.

5. Take it out of the oven when ready. Chill before serving.

Parmesan Crisps[20]

Total time: 20 minutes

Number of servings: 2

Ingredients

- 8 tablespoons grated Parmesan cheese

- 2 slices provolone cheese

- 1 medium jalapeno

Instructions

1. On a baking paper, put 8 mounds of Parmesan cheese, keeping an inch distance from one another.

2. Slice the jalapeno and place it on the baking paper. Cook it at 425 °F for approximately 5 minutes.

3. Take it out of the oven. Allow to chill and then place each one onto a mound of Parmesan. Also, press it down slightly.

4. Divide each provolone slice into pieces and then put them over jalapeno and Parmesan.

5. Let it cook for another 5 minutes. After that, take it out and allow to chill.

6. Serve and enjoy.

---

[20] Volia, I. (n.d.). Mediterranean diet for beginners: With over 120 best healthy food recipes, meal plan to lose weight. Independently Published, p. 124.

Garlic Bread

Total time: 1 hour

Number of servings: 4

Ingredients

- 3 pieces egg white
- 2 teaspoons apple cider vinegar
- 1 teaspoon sea salt
- 300 milliliters almond flour
- 5 tablespoons ground psyllium husk powder
- 2 teaspoons baking powder
- 300 milliliters boiling water
- garlic butter
- 110 grams butter
- 1 garlic clove
- 2 teaspoons chopped fresh parsley
- salt

Instructions

1. Mix the dry ingredients in a bowl and preheat the oven at 350 °F.

2. Boil the water. Add egg whites and vinegar to the bowl and then stir or whisk for 30 seconds using a mixer, but

make sure you don't over mix.

3. Using your hands, make 10 pieces, rolling them into hot dog buns. Create enough space on the baking sheet to enable expansion.

4. Place in the oven on lower rack and leave to bake for 50 minutes.

5. Prepare garlic butter as the bread is baking by mixing all ingredients together. Next, place it in the fridge.

6. Remove the buns from the oven and let them cool. Remove the garlic butter from the fridge and set aside.

7. Slice the buns in halves and spread the garlic butter on each side and then proceed to bake the bread for 10 minutes.

Chocolate Biscuits

Total time: 25 minutes

Number of servings: 8

Ingredients

- 2 cups whole almonds
- 2 tablespoons chia seeds
- ¼ cup unsweetened shredded coconut
- 1 egg
- 1 cup coconut oil
- ¼ cup cocoa powder
- 3 tablespoons stevia
- ¼ teaspoon salt
- 1 teaspoon baking soda

Instructions

1. Preheat the oven at 350 °F.

2. Mix chia seeds and whole almonds into a very fine mixture.

3. Mix all the ingredients together.

4. Cover the mixture with aluminum foil and refrigerate it for 30 minutes.

5. Cut the dough so that you have many thin biscotti

shapes and then leave it to bake for approximately 12 minutes.

6. You can serve it warm or after the dessert has cooled.

Zucchini Chips[21]

Total time: 25 minutes

Number of servings: 4

Ingredients

- 1 pound organic zucchini

- ⅓ cup olive oil

- unrefined sea salt to taste

Instructions

1. Trim the ends of zucchini and then thinly slice them.

2. Oil a microwave-safe plate with olive oil and then place zucchini slices. Spray with olive oil and unrefined sea salt to taste.

3. Cook for 10 minutes uncovered. Check the chips. Cook for more minutes until crispy.

4. Allow to cool and then serve with dressings and dips of your choice.

---

[21] Volia, I. (n.d.). Mediterranean diet for beginners: With over 120 best healthy food recipes, meal plan to lose weight. Independently Published, p. 130.

Tomato and Basil Finger Sandwiches

Total time: 15 minutes

Number of servings: 4

Ingredients

- 4 slices whole-wheat bread

- 8 teaspoons mayonnaise

- 4 thick slices tomatoes

- ⅛ teaspoon freshly ground pepper

- ⅛ teaspoon salt

- 4 teaspoons sliced fresh basil

Instructions

1. Make sure you slice the bread into pieces that are larger than the tomatoes and then put mayonnaise on each slice.

2. Top it with pepper, basil, salt, and tomatoes.

Pepperoni Chips[22]

Total time: 20 minutes

Number of servings: 4

Ingredient

- 4 ounces pepperoni

Instructions

1. Turn the oven to broil and then line the baking sheet with parchment paper.

2. Place pepperoni slices in a single layer. Bake for 2 minutes and watch as they brown in the edges.

3. Remove from the oven. Transfer to a tray and allow to cool for 10 minutes.

4. Serve and enjoy.

---

[22] Volia, I. (n.d.). Mediterranean diet for beginners: With over 120 best healthy food recipes, meal plan to lose weight. Independently Published, p. 128.

Stuffed Celery Bites[23]

Ingredients

- olive oil cooking spray
- 1 minced garlic clove
- 2 tablespoons pine nuts
- 8 stalks celery
- celery leaves
- ¼ cup shredded Italian cheese blend
- 1 piece (8 ounces) fat-free cream cheese
- 2 tablespoons dry-roasted sunflower seeds

Directions

1. Coat a nonstick pan using olive oil cooking spray. Add pine nuts and garlic and then sauté at medium heat for approximately 4 minutes or until you notice the nuts to be golden brown.

2. Put aside.

3. Cut off the wide base and tops from celery and remove 2 thin strips from the round side of celery to create a flat surface.

---

[23] McDonell, L. (2016). The Mediterranean diet for beginners: 110 delicious recipes and the complete guide to going Mediterranean. Independently Published, p. 261.

4. Combine Italian cheese and cream cheese in a bowl. Spread into celery and cut each celery stalk into 2-inch pieces.

5. Sprinkle half of the celery pieces with sunflower seeds and half with the pine nut mixture. Cover and let stand for at least 4 hours before serving.

Healthy Nachos

This type of snack can be prepared very easy and fast. It takes around 10 minutes to prepare the ingredients and just 2 minutes to cook, leading to a total of 12 minutes. In the end, you should have portions for 6 persons. Speaking of ingredients, you can find them below.

Ingredients

- 1 medium thinly sliced green onion
- 1 drained and finely chopped plum tomato
- 2 teaspoons sun-dried tomatoes oil from a container
- 2 tablespoons finely chopped sun-dried tomatoes in oil
- 2 tablespoons finely chopped Kalamata olives
- 4 ounce of restaurant-style corn tortilla chips
- 1 package (4 ounces) finely crumbled feta cheese

Directions

1. Add in a small bowl sun-dried tomatoes, the plum tomato, olives, the onion, and the oil, and then mix them all together. Place aside.

2. Put the tortillas chips in a single layer on a plate and then add cheese on top (evenly). Microwave the whole thing for 1 minute.

3. Change the position of the plate and then microwave it for approximately 30 seconds or until you notice the cheese to be bubbly.

4. Spread the tomato mixture evenly over the cheese and tomatoes. Serve immediately.

Jalapeno Boats

Ingredients

- 1 bag (12 ounces) vegetarian burger crumbles

- 1 cup shredded Parmesan cheese

- 1 package (8 ounces) softened light cream cheese

- 22 large jalapeno peppers, cut into halves lengthwise with the seeds removed

Directions

1. Use a large pan to sauté crumbles over medium heat for approximately 5 minutes or until heated properly.

2. In a small bowl, mix together softened cream cheese and Parmesan cheese, and then fold in the crumble.

3. Let the oven preheat at 425 °F. Take 1 tablespoon out of the crumble-cheese mixture and add it into each jalapeno half. Place the jalapeno halves with the cheese side up on a parchment paper and let it bake in the preheated oven for approximately 20 minutes or until the filling is lightly browned and bubbly.

Roasted Veggie Hummus

Preparing a homemade hummus can be very challenging, but if you follow this recipe, you should get a very delicious snack. The whole process should last for about an hour, with 20 minutes as preparation time and 40 minutes as cooking time. In the end, you should have enough hummus for 20 servings. Below you can find the ingredients for this delicious snack.

Ingredients

- 1 bulb garlic
- ¾ cup olive oil
- 1 halved eggplant
- 1 halved red bell pepper
- ⅓ cup freshly squeezed lemon juice
- 2 cans chickpeas (drained)
- ¼ cup sesame tahini paste
- ⅓ teaspoon smoked paprika
- ½ teaspoon salt

Direction

1. Prepare the oven at 450 °F and place foil over a baking tray.

2. Take out the top of the garlic bulb and put 1 teaspoon of olive oil on it.

3. Wrap the garlic bulb in foil.

4. Add the bell pepper and the eggplant on a different pan. Add 2 tablespoons of olive oil and mix them all together until they are properly coated.

5. Put the wrapped garlic in the pan with the rest of the veggies.

6. Place the wrapped garlic into the pan containing the vegetables.

7. Let them roast for approximately 30 minutes without covering the tray, and when ready, let it cool for around 10 minutes.

8. Take the peels of the bell pepper and eggplant and slice the veggies into small chunks.

9. Put the chickpeas in a food processor and blend them until you get a smooth mixture.

10. Squeeze the pulp from the garlic into the food processor and then place all the ingredients in the food processor. Process them until they are properly mixed.

11. Put the mixture into small serving bowls. You can refrigerate them or serve immediately.

Pesto Stuffed Mushrooms[24]

How long are you willing to spend in order to prepare a healthy snack? Are you willing to spend more than six hours? The mushrooms required for this snack have to be dehydrated, a process that takes around 6 hours. Also, it involves an extra 15 minutes to prepare the ingredients. Speaking of ingredients, you can find them below.

Ingredients

- 14+ button mushrooms, stemmed and washed
- ½ cup extra virgin olive oil
- 3 garlic cloves
- 2 cups basil
- ½ cup pine nuts
- 1 cup walnuts
- ½ teaspoon sea salt

Directions

1. Arrange the mushroom caps top-side down on a plate.
2. In a food processor, blend together stuffing ingredients until very smooth.

---

24 McDonell, L. (2016). The Mediterranean diet for beginners: 110 delicious recipes and the complete guide to going Mediterranean. Independently Published, p. 262.

3. Scoop an equal amount of the stuffing into each cap and dehydrate at 105 °F until soft (about 6 hours).

4. Serve warm.

Chapter 10: Dinner

Dinner is very important in the Mediterranean diet. Your last meal of the day should be in style. While normal diets impose a restriction on calorie intake, this diet doesn't mention anything about consuming fewer calories. However, this doesn't mean that you have to eat more than ever at dinner. As you are about to sleep in a few hours, you don't want to give the digestive system too much work in the evening or during your sleep. The recipes below are well balanced and not that dense in calories. So in order to end your day in style, you may need to choose from any of the meals below.

Mediterranean Stuffed Chicken

Total time: 25 minutes

Number of servings: 2

Ingredients

- 4 boneless and skinless chicken breast halves (or 1½ pounds)

- ¼ cup crumbled reduced feta cheese

- 2 tablespoons finely chopped roasted red sweet peppers

- 15 ounces roasted bell peppers

- 2 tablespoons thinly sliced green onion

- 2 tablespoons snipped fresh oregano

- ½ teaspoon crushed dried oregano

- ½ teaspoon ground black pepper

Instructions

1. Cut a pocket in all 4 chicken breasts using a sharp knife. Aim for the thickest part. Put aside the chicken breast.

2. In a bowl, mix together the green onion, roasted peppers, oregano, and the feta cheese. Stuff the chicken breast pockets with this mixture and then spice them with some black pepper.

3. Put the chicken breast in a pan over medium heat. Let it cook for approximately 15 minutes or until you notice the meat turning white (from pink). While cooking, the

temperature of the thickest part should be 170 °F.

4. As for grilling instructions, put the chicken on the rack and let it grill without being covered for about 15 minutes at medium heat. Flip over the chicken breast halfway through and let it grill for 10 more additional minutes.

5. Let it cool and then serve.

Pan-Roasted with Apples and Brussels Sprouts

Total time: 30 minutes

Number of servings: 3

Ingredients

- 4 chicken thighs or 2 pounds of it

- 1 pound of fresh Brussels sprouts

- 1 thinly sliced medium apple

- 3 tablespoon maple syrup

- 1 teaspoon snipped fresh thyme

Instructions

1. Remove the skin from the chicken thighs and spice them with salt and ground black pepper.

2. Pour some olive oil into a pan. Let it heat at medium flame and then put the chicken thighs into the pan. Let it cook for approximately 10 minutes or until you notice them turning crisp or brown.

3. Flip them once. Partially cover them and let them cook for another 15 minutes at medium heat or until the inside temperature reaches 170 °F. Take the chicken out of the pan and then allow them to stay warm.

4. Prepare the Brussels sprouts by trimming and removing the outer leaves. Wash and drain them properly. Place

the Brussels sprouts into the hot pan and cook them for 5 minutes. At this point, add the apples. Cover the pan and cook for 5 minutes or until the sprouts become tender and golden. (You will have to stir occasionally.) Sprinkle some maple syrup over it and then mix everything together to coat.

5. Transfer the apples and Brussels sprouts into a platter and then place the chicken thighs on top and drizzle some thyme. Serve and enjoy!

Chorizo and Chicken Tray Bake[25]

Total time: 1 hour 55 minutes

Number of servings: 4

Ingredients

- 8 chicken thigh fillets

- 180 grams marinated Kalamata olives

- 200 grams sliced chorizo

- 6 small rosemary sprigs

- 1 lemon, cut into wedges

Instructions

1. Get the oven preheated to 350 °F and then rinse the chicken and pat dry.

2. Place the chicken on a baking tray in a single layer alongside lemon wedges and the fresh rosemary sprigs.

3. Pour reserved olive marinade over the chicken and then pop it into the oven and cook for about 30 minutes.

4. Add chorizo and olives to the pan. Bake for 15 more minutes or until the chicken is well cooked through.

5. Serve with preferred salad, pasta, or rice.

---

[25] Volia, I. (n.d.). Mediterranean diet for beginners: With over 120 best healthy food recipes, meal plan to lose weight. Independently Published.

Salmon with Chili Lime

Total time: 15 minutes

Number of servings: 2

Ingredients

For the steaming salmon:

- 5 ounces salmon fillets
- freshly ground black pepper (to taste)
- sea salt
- 1 cup of water

For the chili lime sauce:

- 1 diced jalapeno seeds
- 1 juiced lime
- 2 minced cloves garlic
- 1 tablespoon honey
- 1 tablespoon olive oil
- 1 tablespoon chopped fresh parsley
- ½ tablespoon cumin
- ½ teaspoon paprika
- 1 tablespoon hot water

Instructions

1. Mix all the ingredients for the sauce into a bowl, and then put aside.

2. Pour some water into the pot and then put the salmon fillets on top of the steam rack in the pot.

3. Use salt and pepper to season the salmon. Cover the pot with a lid and then lock.

4. On steam mode, cook it at high pressure for about 5 minutes.

5. Once the salmon is cooked, just use the quick release method to end the cooking.

6. Place the salmon into a serving plate. Sprinkle some chili lime sauce over it.

7. Serve and enjoy.

Veggie and Mahi-Mahi Skillet[26]

Total time: 30 minutes

Number of servings: 4

Ingredients

- 3 tablespoons olive oil
- 4 mahi-mahi (6 ounces each)
- ½ pound baby portobello mushrooms
- 3 sweet red peppers
- 1 large sweet onion
- ⅓ cup lemon juice
- ¾ teaspoon salt
- ½ teaspoon pepper
- ⅓ cup pine nuts

Instructions

1. Place a skillet over medium heat and then add 2 tablespoons of olive oil. Add fillets and cook for 5 minutes on each side until the fish begins to flake easily with a fork. After that, remove from the pan.
2. Add the remaining oil, peppers, onion, mushrooms,

---

[26] Volia, I. (n.d.). Mediterranean diet for beginners: With over 120 best healthy food recipes, meal plan to lose weight. Independently Published.

lemon juice, and ¼ teaspoon of salt into the pan. Cook while covered for 8 minutes or until the vegetables are tender.

3. Place the fish over the vegetables and then sprinkle with the remaining salt and pepper. Cook for about 2 minutes while covered or until heated through. Sprinkle with chives and pine nuts before serving.

Sautéed Pork Chops with Garlic Spinach

Total time: 20 minutes

Number of servings: 4

Ingredients

- 2 tablespoons olive oil

- 4 bone-in pork loin chops (or 8 ounces)

- ¼ teaspoon salt and pepper

- 1 lemon

- 3 garlic cloves, thinly sliced

- 2 packages fresh spinach (stems removed)

Instructions

1. Put a large pot at medium heat. Pour some oil into it and then heat. Spice the pork chops with pepper and salt and then put them into the pot. Fry for about 5 minutes on each side.

2. Take the pork chops out of the pot and then put them on a platter. Sprinkle the lemon juice over them. Cover the chops with foil and then allow approximately 5 minutes to cool before serving.

3. In order to cook the garlic spinach, put a pot over medium heat, pour some oil into it, and heat. Put garlic and cook for approximately 30 seconds or until fragrant. Add spinach into the pot and cook for approximately 3 minutes or until wilted.

4. Spice it with salt and pepper and then stir. Take it out from the heat. Pour some lemon juice on it.

5. Place it into a platter. Take the foil from the pork chops and serve them garnished with the garlic spinach.

Kale, Potato, and Bacon Frittata

Total time: 30 minutes

Number of servings: 6

Ingredients

- 12 ounces tiny red new potatoes
- less-fat bacon, coarsely chopped with lower sodium
- 2 cups freshly chopped kale
- 1 medium chopped onion
- eggs, lightly beaten

Instructions

1. Put a saucepan at medium heat and then pour water and add salt. Put in the potatoes, cover them, and cook for about 10 minutes or until you notice the potatoes to be tender. Drain them and place aside.

2. Preheat the broiler. In a large pot, cook the bacon over medium heat until it is crisp. Add kale and onion and then cook for about 5 minutes. Stir the cooked potatoes.

3. In a bowl, whisk the salt, ground black pepper, and eggs and cook the eggs mixture over low heat. As the mixture starts to fry, use a rubber spatula around the edges to lift the egg mixture in order for the uncooked portion to go underneath and get cooked.

4. Continue to cook and lift the edges until the egg mixture is ready. After that, put the pot under the broiler and make sure it is about 5 inches from heat.

5. Broil it for approximately 2 minutes or until the top is well cooked, dried, and no longer wet. Preheat the oven at 400 °F and then leave it to bake for about 5 minutes.

6. Let it cool for approximately 5 minutes. After that, place the frittata onto a serving platter.

Cumin Thyme Granola with Roasted Carrots[27]

Total time: 30 minutes

Number of servings: 4

Ingredients

- 1½ pounds carrots

- 1 tablespoon olive oil

- ¼ teaspoon salt and pepper

- 1 tablespoon lemon juice

- ½ finely chopped shallot

- 1 teaspoon fresh thyme leaves

- 1 cup thyme granola

Instructions

1. On a rimmed baking dish, toss the carrots with olive oil, salt, and pepper.

2. Set the oven to 400 °F and then bake for 25 minutes or until tender and golden brown.

3. In a bowl, mix the lemon juice with a teaspoon of olive

---

[27] Volia, I. (n.d.). Mediterranean diet for beginners: With over 120 best healthy food recipes, meal plan to lose weight. Independently Published.

oil, fresh thyme leaves, finely chopped shallot, and a teaspoon of salt and pepper.

4. Drizzle the mixture over carrots and then sprinkle with thyme granola.

5. Serve and enjoy.

Citrus Scallops[28]

Total time: 15 minutes

Number of servings: 4

Ingredients

- 1 medium red or green pepper, julienned

- 4 chopped green onions

- 1 minced garlic clove

- 2 tablespoons olive oil

- 1 pound sea scallops

- ¼ teaspoon crushed red pepper flakes

- 2 tablespoons lime juice

- ½ teaspoon grated lime zest

- 4 medium oranges

- 2 teaspoons minced fresh cilantro

- hot cooked rice pasta

---

[28] Volia, I. (n.d.). Mediterranean diet for beginners: With over 120 best healthy food recipes, meal plan to lose weight. Independently Published.

Instructions

1. Place a skillet over medium heat and then add oil and heat. Sauté garlic for 30 seconds. Add onions and pepper. Cook for about 3 minutes.

2. Add lime juice and zest. Cook for a minute and reduce heat. Add orange sections and cilantro. Cook for two more minutes until the scallops become opaque.

3. Serve with pasta, rice, or your preferred dish.

Mediterranean Chicken Made Easy

Total time: 25 minutes

Number of servings: 4

Ingredients

- 4 boneless chicken breasts (or 5 ounces)
- ¼ cup freshly chopped basil
- 1 tablespoon olive oil
- halved cherry tomatoes
- ¼ cup olive tapenade
- ¼ teaspoon sea salt

Instructions

1. Grease a baking tray and place the chicken breast in it. Season it with 2 tablespoons of basil and salt. Use parchment paper to cover the baking tray.

2. Put a frying pan at medium heat and then pour some oil into it. Fry the chicken breasts for approximately 6 minutes on each side until they get browned.

3. Take the chicken breast out of the pan once it is cooked and then wrap it in aluminum foil to keep warm.

4. Put olive tapenade and tomatoes into the same pan and then cook for about 3 minutes.

5. Place the chicken into a platter and then pour on it the tomato and tapenade mixture. Use the remaining basil to season and enjoy.

Cashew Beef Thai Stir-Fry

Total time: 40 minutes

Number of servings: 2

Ingredients

- 2 tablespoons toasted sesame seed oil
- 2 garlic cloves
- 1 teaspoon ginger
- 1 carrot
- ¼ medium red onion
- 1 zucchini
- 1 jalapeno
- 1 pound beef
- salt and pepper (to taste)
- ¼ teaspoon red pepper flakes
- ¼ teaspoon Chinese five-spice
- ¼ cup beef broth
- ¼ cup coconut milk
- 1 ounce cashews
- 1 bunch fresh basil

Instructions

1. Mince the garlic and then slice and chop all vegetables.

2. Put a pot at medium heat and then pour sesame seed oil. Put in carrots, onion, ginger, and garlic. Cook them until they become fragrant.

3. Season with zucchini and jalapenos and then mix them all together. Place aside.

4. Slice the beef thinly and then pour some toasted sesame oil into a skillet. Fry the beef until it turns brown on all sides.

5. Spice the beef with Chinese five-spice pepper, red pepper flakes, and salt.

6. Put in the veggies to the browned beef and then stir. At this point, pour the beef broth and coconut milk. You can also add heavy cream.

7. Put in some cashews and cook it for approximately 8 minutes.

8. Add some fresh basil into the pot. Stir and mix. Cook it for 5 additional minutes.

9. Use a green onion to garnish, then serve.

Sweet-Chili Salmon with Blackberries[29]

Total time: 25 minutes

Number of servings: 4

Ingredients

- 1 cup frozen blackberries, thawed
- 1 cup finely chopped cucumbers
- 1 green onion, finely chopped
- 2 tablespoons of sweet chili sauce
- 4 salmon fillets (6 ounces each)
- ½ teaspoon salt and pepper

Instructions

1. In a bowl, combine the cucumber, blackberries, green onion, and 1 teaspoon of chili sauce and then toss to coat.

2. Sprinkle salmon with salt and pepper. After that, place it on a greased grill rack. Grill the fillet while covered over medium heat or broil for 12 minutes from heat or until the fish easily flakes with a fork.

3. Brush with the remaining chili sauce in the last 3 minutes of cooking.

4. Serve with some blackberry mixture.

---

[29] Volia, I. (n.d.). Mediterranean diet for beginners: With over 120 best healthy food recipes, meal plan to lose weight. Independently Published.

Curried Chicken with Cauliflower, Apricots, and Olives

Total time: 8 hours 50 minutes

Refrigerator time: 8 hours

Prep time: 15 minutes

Cooking time: 35 minutes

Yield: 4 to 6 servings

Ingredients

- 8 chicken thighs, boneless and skinless

- ¼ cup extra-virgin olive oil

- ½ teaspoon ground cinnamon

- ¼ teaspoon cayenne pepper

- 1 teaspoon smoked paprika

- 4 teaspoons curry powder

- 1 tablespoon apple cider vinegar

- sea salt (to taste)

- 1 chopped head cauliflower

- 1 cup halved pitted green olives

- ¾ cup chop and dried apricots, soaked in hot water, drained

- ⅓ cup chopped fresh cilantro

- 6 lemon wedges

Directions

1. In a medium bowl, mix sea salt, vinegar, curry powder, ½ teaspoon of paprika, cayenne, cinnamon, 2 tablespoons of extra-virgin oil with the chicken thighs. Toss them together to coat. Cover them and refrigerate for approximately 8 hours.

2. Place a rack in the center of the oven and then preheat the oven at 450 °F.

3. Place some parchment paper in a pan. Add the remaining olive oil, curry powder, paprika, and cauliflower. Mix them properly.

4. Add apricots and olive, then spread the mixture into a single layer.

5. Just over the cauliflower mixture, place the chicken thighs, with even space between them. Roast them in the oven for approximately 35 minutes or until cauliflower is brown and the chicken is properly cooked.

6. Sprinkle cilantro over the cauliflower and chicken and garnish it with lemon wedges.

Penne with Chicken[30]

Total time: 50 minutes

Prep time: 20 minutes

Cooking time: 30 minutes

Yield: 4 servings

Ingredients

- 1 package pasta (penne)
- 1½ tablespoons butter
- ½ cup chopped red onion
- 2 minced garlic cloves
- ¾ kilogram chicken breasts, halved and skinned
- 1 can artichoke hearts, chopped and soaked in water
- ½ cup crumbled feta cheese
- 2 tablespoons lemon juice
- 1 chopped tomato
- 3 tablespoons fresh parsley
- sea salt

---

[30] McDonell, L. (2016). The Mediterranean diet for beginners: 110 delicious recipes and the complete guide to going Mediterranean. Independently Published.

- black pepper (freshly ground)

- 1 teaspoon dried oregano

Directions

1. In a large pot boil some water, add salt into it. When it is *al dente*, put the penne pasta in to boil (check the instructions on the package to find out for how many minutes you have to boil this pasta).

2. Heat a large skillet over medium flame. Melt butter into it, and then add the garlic and onions.

3. Cook them for about 2 minutes and then add the chicken.

4. Stir occasionally for about 6 minutes until you notice the chicken to get golden brown.

5. Add the artichoke hearts to the skillet after draining them, together with the drained pasta, parsley, oregano, tomatoes, lemon juice, and cheese.

6. Lower the heat to medium-low and let it cook for approximately 3 minutes.

7. Add pepper and salt to taste (if needed) and serve warm.

Parmesan Meatloaf

Total time: 1 hour

Prep time: 10 minutes

Cook time: 50 minutes

Yield: 4 servings

Ingredients

- 1½ pounds ground beef
- ½ cup bread crumbs
- ½ cup parsley leaves, chopped flat
- 1 grated onion
- 1 large egg
- ½ cup grated Parmesan
- ¼ cup tomato paste
- Sea salt
- black pepper, freshly ground

Directions

1. Preheat your oven to 400 °F. In a large bowl, mix together ground beef, bread crumbs, parsley, onion, egg, Parmesan cheese, tomato paste, sea salt, and pepper.

2. Line a baking sheet with foil and add the beef mixture, pressing to form an 8-inch loaf.

3. Bake in the preheated oven for about 50 minutes or until cooked through.

Fish with Olives, Tomatoes, and Capers

Total time: 21 minutes

Prep time: 5 minutes

Cook time: 16 minutes

Yield: 4 servings

Ingredients

- 4 teaspoons extra-virgin olive oil

- 4 sea bass fillets (5 ounces)

- 1 small onion, diced

- ½ cup white wine

- 2 tablespoon capers

- 1 cup canned tomatoes, diced and with juice

- ½ cup chopped pitted black olives

- ¼ teaspoon crushed red pepper

- 2 cups fresh baby spinach leaves

- sea salt and pepper

Directions

1. Use a large pot to heat some extra-virgin olive oil (about 2 teaspoons) at medium-high heat.

2. Put the fish in and fry it for about 3 minutes per each side.

3. Take the cooked fish out of the pot and into a plate and keep it warm.

4. Pour the remaining oil into the pot and fry the onion for approximately 2 minutes.

5. Pour in the wine and cook for 2 more minutes or until the liquid is decreased to half.

6. Add in the red pepper, olives, tomatoes, and capers and cook them all together for approximately 3 more minutes.

7. Put the spinach in, cook it, and make sure you stir it for approximately 3 minutes or until it gets wilted.

8. Add some pepper and salt, and pour the sauce over the fish.

9. Serve immediately.

Pasta with Shrimp

Total time: 20 minutes

Prep time: 15 minutes

Cooking time: 5 minutes

Yield: 4 servings

Ingredients

- 2 teaspoons extra-virgin olive oil
- 2 minced garlic cloves
- 1 pound peeled and deveined shrimp
- 2 cups chopped plum tomato
- ¼ cup fresh basil, thinly sliced
- 2 tablespoons drained capers
- ⅓ cup pitted Kalamata olives, chopped
- ¼ teaspoon of black pepper, freshly ground
- 4 cups angel hair pasta, hot cooked
- ¼ cup feta cheese, crumbled
- cooking spray

Directions

1. Use a large pot and heat it at medium-high flame. Pour some extra-virgin olive oil and let it heat. Add the garlic and cook it for about 30 seconds.

2. Put in the shrimp and fry it for approximately 1 minute.

3. Add the basil and tomato. Stir them, and then decrease the heat to medium-low. Cook them for approximately 3 minutes or until you notice the tomato is tender.

4. Add black peppers, the Kalamata olives, and the capers.

5. In a large bowl, combine the shrimp mixture with pasta. Stir to mix them all together and sprinkle some cheese on top.

6. Serve immediately.

Chapter 11: Dessert

Rustic Almond and Pear Cake

Ingredients

- 1 cup almond meal
- 2 cups plain flour
- ½ teaspoon ground cardamom
- ¼ teaspoon ground cinnamon
- 1 teaspoon vanilla essence
- 1½ teaspoon baking powder
- ¼ teaspoon coarse sea salt
- 3 eggs
- 4 tablespoons full-fat Greek yogurt
- ½ cup coconut oil
- ½ cup olive oil
- 2 tablespoons honey
- 1 cup of brown sugar
- 3 pears, peeled, chopped, and cored
- ½ cup soaked cranberries
- 4 tablespoons chopped almonds

Sauce:

- ½ cup melted stick butter

- ¾ cup brown sugar

- ⅓ cup double cream

Directions

1. Thoroughly mix the baking powder, vanilla, salt, cardamom, cinnamon, plain flour, and almond meal until everything is properly incorporated.

2. Then beat the Greek yogurt and eggs using an electric mixer until frothy. Add the olive and coconut oil and blend to mix well. Stir in the sugar and honey and blend again.

3. Add now the wet ingredients on the dry mixture and blend again. Fold in the chopped almonds, cranberries, and pears.

4. Put your batter into a lightly greased pan. Leave it to bake in the oven at 360 °F for approximately 35 minutes. To verify if it is done, use a tester and insert it in the middle of the cake.

5. In the meantime, melt the butter in a pan at low heat. Now, stir in the double cream and brown sugar. Leave it to cook until you see the caramel starting to boil.

6. Cut the cake into slices and add some caramel sauce over it. Bon appétit!

Almond Shortbread Cookies

Ingredients

- 1 cup powdered sugar

- ½ cup coconut oil

- ½ cup butter (kept at room temperature)

- 2 egg yolks

- 1 tablespoon rose flower water

- 1 tablespoon brandy

- 1 teaspoon vanilla extract

- 3½ cups cake flour

- 1 cup finely ground blanched almonds

Cooking Instructions

1. Blend the softened butter, coconut oil, and powdered sugar using an electric mixer on high speed.

2. Add in the vanilla extract, brandy, rose flower water, and egg yolks. Blend again to combine.

3. Put in the almonds and flour and then stir using a wooden spoon. You need to leave the whole thing in your refrigerator for about 1 hour and 30 minutes.

4. In the meantime, heat the oven to 325 °F. Use your hands to shape the dough into 1-inch balls and place them on a baking sheet. Make sure you flatten each ball.

5. Bake the cookies in the preheated oven for approximately 10 to 13 minutes or until they are ready. Take your cookies out of the oven and leave them to cool before serving. Enjoy!

Homemade Halvah with Walnuts[31]

Ingredients

- ¼ cup water (kept at room temperature)
- ⅓ cup powdered sugar
- 2 tablespoons golden syrup (light treacle)
- 3 tablespoons ghee
- 1 teaspoon vanilla powder
- ¾ cup sesame paste (tahini)
- ½ cup roughly chopped walnuts
- ⅛ teaspoon ground cinnamon
- ¼ teaspoon freshly grated nutmeg
- ¼ teaspoon sea salt
- 1 teaspoon freshly squeezed lemon juice

Cooking Instructions

1. Lightly spritz a 9-inch pan with a nonstick cooking spray.

2. Boil the water and sugar in a medium saucepan over medium-high heat. Immediately reduce the heat and

[31] Thornton, A. (2019). Mediterranean diet cookbook for beginners: Easy and healthy Mediterranean recipes for weight loss. Independently Published.

cook for 15 minutes until the liquid coats a spoon thickly. Fold in the golden syrup.

3. Mix the remaining ingredients until well combined. Fold in the sugar syrup and stir quickly until everything is uniform.

4. Pour the batter into the prepared pan. Press down with a spatula.

5. Allow it to cool down completely. After that, cover it with plastic wrap and refrigerate for at least 24 hours. Cut the cold halvah into slices or cubes and serve.

Poached Peaches with Blue Cheese Cream[32]

Ingredients

- ¼ teaspoon cardamom pods
- 1 cinnamon stick
- 1 vanilla bean
- 3 whole cloves
- 1 teaspoon allspice berries
- ⅓ cup orange juice
- 1 teaspoon orange zest
- ⅔ cup red wine
- 4 peaches
- 4 ounces sliced blue cheese, sliced
- 4 tablespoons dried cherries
- 2 tablespoons Greek honey

Directions

1. Add the cardamom, cinnamon, vanilla, cloves, allspice, orange juice, orange zest, and red wine to a deep saucepan.

---

[32] Thornton, A. (2019). Mediterranean diet cookbook for beginners: Easy and healthy Mediterranean recipes for weight loss. Independently Published.

2. Add your peaches and poach them for 2 hours or until they have softened. Remove the peaches with a slotted spoon. To make a syrup, boil the leftover liquid until it reduces by half.

3. In the meantime, mix the blue cheese, dried cherries, and honey. Slice your peaches into halves; top each peach with the blue cheese cream. Drizzle with some extra syrup and serve immediately. Enjoy!

Greek Loukoumades with Chocolate Sauce

Ingredients

Dough:

- 2 cups all-purpose flour
- a pinch of sea salt
- 1 teaspoon brown sugar
- 1½ ounce active dry yeast
- 2 beaten eggs
- ½ cup warm full-fat milk
- 1 cup warm water
- ½ teaspoon vanilla extract

Chocolate sauce:

- 2 ounces water
- 2 ounces caster sugar
- 6 ounces dark chocolate chunks

Directions

1. Put the flour and mix in a pinch of salt. In a mixing bowl, whisk ½ cup of water, yeast, and brown sugar. You will have to whisk until the yeast dissolves completely.

2. Put in the remaining ingredients for the dough and whisk at high speed for approximately 1 to 2 minutes.

3. Cover the whole thing with plastic wrap. Keep the dough in a warm place for more than 1 hour in order to rise.

4. Use a frying pan to properly fry the loukoumades (pour plenty of cooking oil). When the oil is sizzling, you can fry your loukoumades, one batch at a time.

5. During the frying process, press them into the oil to make sure they fry on all sides until they are slightly brown. Take your loukoumades out of the frying pan and place them on a kitchen paper to drain. Repeat the process with the remaining dough.

6. In a different saucepan, cook the water and sugar for about 1–2 minutes or until the sugar is completely dissolved. Add the chocolate and blend until the chocolate is completely melted.

7. Using a spoon, put the warm chocolate over your loukoumades and enjoy!

Grilled Pineapple with Mint and Strawberries[33]

Total Time: 30 minutes

Number of servings: 4

Ingredients

- 1 pineapple

- ¼ cup olive oil

- 3 tablespoons honey

- 2 teaspoons sriracha chili sauce

- 1 cup sliced strawberries

- ½ teaspoon salt

- mint leaves for garnish

- ice cream

Instructions

1. Prepare pineapple marinade by combining olive oil, honey, sriracha, and salt in a bowl and then set aside.

2. Cut pineapple at the top and bottom and then remove the outer skin. Cut pineapple into slices of about ⅜ inch thick and

---

[33] Volia, I. (n.d.). Mediterranean diet for beginners: With over 120 best healthy food recipes, meal plan to lose weight. Independently Published.

then place in a ziplock bag. Pour marinade over them. After that, seal the bag and rub to distribute the marinade.

3. Allow it to marinate for 4 hours. Preheat the grill and then get the pineapples grilled on both sides for about 3 minutes.

4. Transfer the grilled pineapple to a plate. Top with mint leaves and sliced strawberries.

5. Serve with a scoop of ice cream.

No-Bake Cheesecake

Total time: 2 hours

Number of servings: 4

Ingredients

- 4 ounces cream cheese
- 2 tablespoons sour cream
- ¼ cup heavy whipping cream
- ¼ cup of erythritol
- unsweetened Baker's chocolate

Instructions

1. Blend together the whipping cream, sour cream, erythritol, and cream cheese using a hand mixer.

2. Fill in the cupcake molds then put them in the fridge for 2 hours.

Ganache:

1. In the microwave, melt the Baker's chocolate and then add heavy whipping cream. Mix them well.

2. Pour some water over it and then mix until it achieves a thick liquid consistency.

3. Pour it over the frozen cheesecakes and then serve immediately.

Coconut Ice Cream[34]

Total time: 15 minutes

Number of servings: 2

Ingredients

- 15 ounces full-fat coconut milk

- ¾ cup sugar

- a pinch of salt

- 2½ tablespoons cornstarch

- unsweetened shredded coconut, toasted and dried (optional)

Instructions

1. In a saucepan, have all the ingredients combined except for the ¼ cup of coconut milk.

2. Place the saucepan over medium heat and then allow the ingredients to simmer.

3. In a bowl, place cornstarch and the ¼ cup of coconut milk and then whisk together until smooth.

4. Add the cornstarch mixture to the saucepan. After that, allow cooking as you constantly stir until it thickens.

---

[34] Volia, I. (n.d.). Mediterranean diet for beginners: With over 120 best healthy food recipes, meal plan to lose weight. Independently Published.

5. Remove from heat. Allow cooling at room temperature.

6. Cover it up. Allow chilling for about 4 hours.

7. Freeze it in the ice cream maker. Serve with toasted coconut or as desired.

Chocolate Cheese Cake

Total time: 35 minutes

Number of servings: 3

Ingredients

For the crust:

- ¼ cup almond flour
- ¼ cup coconut flour
- 2 tablespoons melted butter
- 2 ½ tablespoons cocoa powder, unsweetened
- low-carb sweetener

For the filling:

- 16 ounces cream cheese
- ½ teaspoon concentrated stevia powder
- ¼ cup sour cream
- 1 egg
- 2 egg yolks
- ⅓ cup cocoa powder
- ½ teaspoon monk fruit powder
- 6 ounces melted baking chocolate
- 1 teaspoons vanilla extract
- ¾ cup heavy cream

Instructions

Crust:

1. Place some parchment paper on a baking tray and make sure it is trimmed to size as it has to fit exactly the bottom of your tray.

2. In a medium-sized bowl, blend all the ingredients for the crust. Add the melted butter, stir, and then place it at the bottom of the baking tray.

Filling:

1. To properly blend the sweeteners, cream cheese, and cocoa powder, you need to use an electric blender.

2. Add in the egg yolks and egg and continue to blend.

3. At this point, add the vanilla extract, melted chocolate, heavy cream, and sour cream. Blend them all together, making sure that all the sides of the bowl remain clean (scrubbing may be necessary).

4. Now that you have a rich mixture, you need to pour it on top of the crust in the baking tray and smoothen everything using a rubber spatula.

5. Add the trivet into the baking tray and then add 2 cups of water.

6. Cover the trivet with a foil and make sure that the ends can be extended to cover the whole top of the tray.

7. Put this cheesecake tray on top of the sling and cover it with the foil to prevent condensation because you will have to fold the sling loosely over the cheesecake.

8. Cover the pot and leave it to cook at high pressure for approximately 20 minutes.

9. For around 10 minutes, release the pressure naturally.

10. Open the lid, lift the cheesecake off, and place it somewhere else to cool, preferably on a cooling rack.

11. You have to let it cool for at least 1 hour and then refrigerate it overnight.

12. Before you serve it, take it out of the refrigerator, let it stay at room temperature for a bit (15 minutes to 30 minutes), and then enjoy it.

Pistachio Pudding

Total time: 30 minutes

Number of servings: 4

Ingredients

- 1 cup shelled unsalted pistachios
- ½ cup granulated sugar
- 2 cups whole milk
- 2 tablespoons of cornstarch
- ¼ cup sugar
- ½ teaspoon salt
- 2 tablespoons unsalted butter
- ¼ tablespoon pure vanilla extract
- whipped cream (to be used for garnish)

Instructions

1. Place the pistachios into a food processor. Blend them for approximately 3 minutes until finely ground. Add 2 tablespoons of milk and ¼ cup of sugar. Blend them all together until you get a paste.

2. Use a saucepan to mix the paste with 2 cups of milk and then place it on the stove at medium heat. While cooking, make sure you whisk them.

3. When the milk is heating up, add salt, cornstarch, egg

yolks, and the remaining sugar into the processor and blend them all together until they are properly mixed.

4. To temper the eggs, just add ½ cup of warm milk into the food processor. Pour the whole mixture from the blender into the pan and make sure you constantly stir to thicken the mixture and then take it off the heat.

5. Add butter and vanilla and stir until the butter melts properly.

6. Split the pudding into 4 serving cups. Cover them with a plastic wrap and let them chill in the refrigerator for around 4 hours.

7. Just before serving, remove them from the refrigerator and top them with whipped cream and chopped pistachios.

Chapter 12: Best Tips
of the Mediterranean Diet

By this chapter, you already realized how healthy this diet is and what its benefits are. If you decide to try it, you need to radically change not only the food you eat but also your lifestyle. Below you can find some valuable tips for switching from the standard Western diet rich in processed and junk food to the Mediterranean, which is rich in healthy fats and suggests better balanced meals in terms of nutritional value.

Switch to Olive Oil

It's widely known that fried food is increasing your cholesterol level dramatically, especially because it is fried in "traditional oil," such as sunflower or vegetable oil. Avoiding fried food is highly recommended, but using olive oil instead of these other oils is among the best thing you can do during this diet. The concentration of healthy fats is exactly what your body needs. Studies have shown that the olive oil can raise the high-density lipoprotein (HDL) cholesterol level, but don't worry about this as HDL is the good type of cholesterol. The low-density lipoprotein (LDL) cholesterol (which by the way is the bad one) is eliminated by the consumption of olive oil. Therefore, you need to use olive oil with most food you eat, whether it is salads, mashed potatoes, or pasta.

Enjoy Eating More Fish

The Mediterranean diet focuses on bringing the right amount of protein and healthy fat. Fish can have the right balance of proteins and fats, and your body can benefit from the consumption of it. Omega-3 fatty acids and other healthy substances can be obtained from consuming fish, like salmon, mackerel, or sardines. Other fish types are also recommended, but it is mandatory to have at least a day of eating fish during your weekly diet. Avoid breading and frying the fish in the "traditional oil" type mentioned above. Use olive oil instead.

Vegetables Should Be a Must on a Daily Basis

There are plenty of vitamins, minerals, and nutrients that can be found in vegetables, so you need to set your daily menu plan, including plenty of vegetables. Every important meal of the day needs to have vegetables, and if you are having snacks, it's recommended that the snack should be based on vegetables. Visit the ingredients chapter to find out more details about the veggies you need to consume.

Stick to Whole Grains

If you do have to eat bread or pasta, stick to whole grains. To get all the benefits of consuming grain, you need to consume them as "whole" as possible because processing grains will lose their nutritional value. The more processed the food type based on grains is, the higher is the carb level. One purpose of the Mediterranean diet should be the lowering of carbs, so try to consume the grains as "whole" as possible. Try to eat bread and pasta from whole grains.

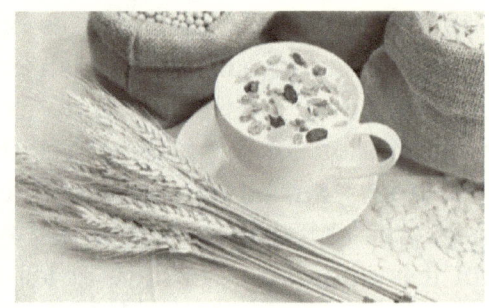

Be "Nuts"

This food type should be on your daily menu, so every time you snack, you need to include nuts, such as pistachios, almonds, cashews, walnuts, and macadamia nuts. Nuts are rich fiber and minerals. If you are low in minerals (e.g., potassium), eating nuts should raise your mineral intake, so you might want to consider this when including nuts in your daily menu.

Eat Fruits

Avoid sweets for dessert and eat fruits instead. Since fruits are rich in vitamins, minerals, antioxidants, and fiber, make sure you include them in your dessert. If you want to add a sweet flavor to your dessert, you might want to use brown sugar or stevia as it is a lot less harmful than normal sugar. If you check chapter 6, you will know exactly what fruits you need to include in your shopping list.

Drink a Bit of Wine

Unlike other diets, the Mediterranean diet encourages the moderate consumption of wine as the body can benefit from the compounds found in a glass of wine. For instance, a glass of red 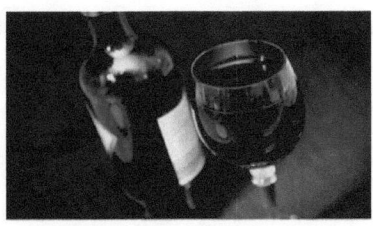 wine can be very good for your blood circulation.

Enjoy Each Bite

Eating on the run will not allow the body to process the food properly. Chewing your food properly will make the job of your digestive system a lot easier. This is how it can process all the nutrients required for the better function of your body. The Mediterranean diet is also more of a lifestyle as it encourages you to take your time when eating. Enjoy your meal with your family and friends. Food is better when you eat it with a nice company.

Plan Your Meals

Plan your meals for a week so that you will know exactly what you need to include in your shopping list. By doing this, you will know exactly when you can eat meat, fish, or pasta.

Make Your Own Dressing

Since the diet emphasizes the consumption of salads a lot, you need to make your own dressing. Sauces bought from supermarkets are not natural, so they may not be recommended when it comes to your salads.

Chapter 13: Mindset Is Important

Having the right attitude toward this diet is very important, as your determination and ambition can only come from your mind. The Mediterranean diet implies a serious number of changes—some of them being more radical than others. As seen in the previous chapter, you need to follow some important rules when being on this diet; otherwise, you're preventing it from delivering the full extent of its benefits.

Your mindset defines who you really are as it represents a collection of opinion and thoughts that are reflected in your attitude. An attitude can be faked but not the mindset. A positive mindset can help you achieve more, so you can also say that it influences your willingness and ambition to achieve your goals through this diet. The Mediterranean diet is a lifestyle, so it's a lot more than a meal plan. This is something you need to stick to for the rest of your life. The change may be radical if you are a big fan of fast food and other forms of processed food, but if you stick to the standard meal plan, most likely, you will end up with obesity or other medical conditions, such as diabetes, heart disease, liver disease, kidney disease, and even different forms of cancer.

Switching to this diet is the normal thing to do to fight against or prevent all the medical conditions or diseases mentioned above. The Mediterranean diet lowers your carb level, as well as your glucose level, forcing your body to run more on fats than glucose. Running on fats is the right thing to do as it is considered the "bio-fuel" the body can run on.

Carbs can be blamed for most of the diseases caused by food, and it also causes addiction. So you need to have a strong will in order to get out of the vicious circle of consuming carbs. It is not something easy to do. Controlling your cravings is a job for your mind, so having the right mindset is extremely important in order to stick to this diet. There are plenty of people who quit their diet because it is too harsh or because they are not motivated enough. These people don't have the right mindset.

This diet should be easy to follow as it doesn't involve too many restrictions. If you plan your meals properly, you can still have food types you thought you couldn't live without a few times per week. However, the diet requires more changes that are not seen at first glance. This book presents all the information you need to know about the Mediterranean diet so that you can decide whether or not you want to try this meal plan/lifestyle. Changes are not easy, especially if you are already used to the same routine, so the mindset can play an essential role in sticking to this diet and respecting all its rules.

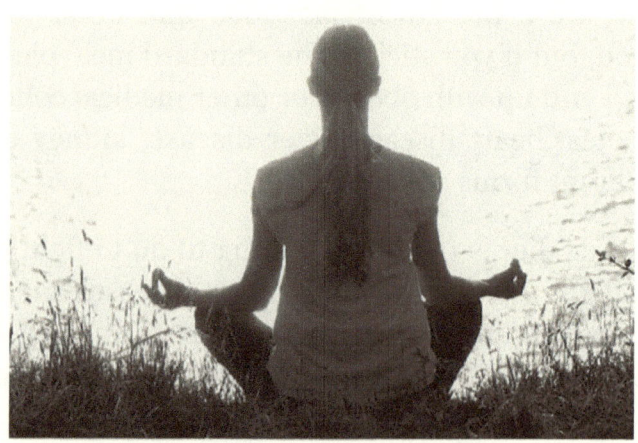

Conclusion

There are too many diseases and medical conditions caused by the food we eat. The quality of food has decreased dramatically over the past decades as the food-processing industry is now providing most of the food we consume. The more processed the food type is, the more harmful it is to your body. For the sake of making profits and processing food in a very efficient manner, food-processing companies are basically providing poison for the consumers.

Finding true organic food is quite difficult as farmers today use all kinds of chemicals to grow crops, fruits, and vegetables while animals are fed with concentrated food to grow at an incredible pace before being slaughtered for meat. All these chemicals used in these types of food are affecting the quality of food and our health. Putting additives to food means processing it even further, but at the same time, it means lowering the quality of food. This has terrible consequences on the human body as it is now being fed with a copious number of carbohydrates.

Processed food is in abundance, and the Western way of life favors the consumption of junk food. This is the reason why obesity and diabetes are becoming very common, especially in the United States and other countries of the Western world. People are now confused and don't know exactly what they should eat since pizza, burgers, and French fries are probably the most common food consumed and sold today. As part of the junk-food category, they have little to no nutritional value. They can provide a temporary sense of satiety, which doesn't last very long. This type of food causes addiction. You will start to feel hungry again, and you will crave for the same type of food.

Not only are junk foods caloric bombs (they are the calorie-dense type of foods), but they also have an incredibly high level of carbohydrates. In such foods, you can find plenty of glucose, which the body uses as an energy source. Energy is obtained by burning the glucose during physical activity, not by eating carbs and gaining more glucose.

Nowadays, people are extremely passive and not very involved in physical activity. That is why using glucose is becoming more of an issue. When not used, the glucose is stored in your blood, raising the insulin and blood sugar level. If the glucose is not used, not enough energy is released. You will constantly feel tired, and most likely, you will not engage in physical activity. This leads to gaining more fat, and eventually, you can get overweight and obese.

A radical change is required, and this is where the Mediterranean diet can make a difference. It is not just a meal plan; it is a lifestyle because you need to try it for a very long time, not just for a few weeks. This diet consists of eating healthy, having a much-diversified menu, and relying more on healthy fats, fruits, and vegetables. The purpose of the diet is to switch the fuel type of the body from glucose to fat—meaning, the body will run on fat.

This metabolic state will favor the fat-burning process and the decrease of insulin and blood sugar level, thus reversing obesity and diabetes. However, this is just the tip of the iceberg when it comes to the health and physical benefits of this diet, as many diseases and health conditions can be prevented or reversed using this diet.

This meal plan is not about restrictions. You can eat a wide variety of food types, and there is no mention of how many calories you need to eat. However, using the recipes provided in this book, you can benefit even more from this diet. You need to remember the Mediterranean diet pyramid. It has at its base physical activity. Therefore, you need to make sure you have an active lifestyle in order to maximize the effects of the Mediterranean diet. Make sure you follow the meal plan for a long time and engage in physical activity (jogging, cycling, swimming, working out, or just playing sports) so that you will experience all the best benefits of this diet.

Bibliography

Cambridge University Press. Retrieved from
www.cambridge.org/core/journals/public-health-
nutrition/article/mediterranean-diet-science-and-
practice/C383082DF00DDFE6475D0B8614EB0BE9

Fernandez, Sonia. (2018) Top 5 Mediterranean diet benefits
backed up by research. Retrieved from
www.medicalnewsbulletin.com/mediterranean-diet-benefits-
research/

Laurence, Emily. (2019). 9 Mediterranean diet benefits that
explain why experts love it so much. Retrieved from
www.wellandgood.com/good-food/mediterranean-diet-
benefits/

McDonell, L. (2016). The Mediterranean diet for beginners:
110 delicious recipes and the complete guide to going
Mediterranean. Independently Published.

Saulle, R. and La Torre, G. (2010). Retrieved from
https://www.researchgate.net/publication/288123570_The_
Mediterranean Diet recognized by UNESCO as a cultural
 heritage of humanity

Thornton, A. (2019). Mediterranean diet cookbook for
beginners: Easy and healthy Mediterranean recipes for weight
loss. Independently Published.

University Health News. (2018). 6 major benefits of the
Mediterranean diet. Retrieved from
www.universityhealthnews.com/daily/nutrition/6-major-
benefits-of-the-mediterranean-diet/

Volia, I. (n.d.). Mediterranean diet for beginners: With over 120 best healthy food recipes, meal plan to lose weight. Independently Published.

Willett, Walter. (2007). The Mediterranean diet: Science and practice. *Cambridge Core*.